CARB CYCLING

DIET GUIDE AND COOKBOOK

FOR WEIGHT LOSS IN WOMEN

A Comprehensive Guide to Low, High, and Moderate Carb Intake for Weight Loss, Hormonal Balance, Muscle Building, Increased Energy, and Craving Control

Judy Kelly

Table of Contents

Introduction

Welcome to the world of Carb Cycling—a flexible and effective approach to not just losing weight, but transforming your relationship with food and your body. If you've ever felt overwhelmed by rigid diets or frustrated by slow progress, you're not alone. Many of us have been on that rollercoaster of dieting highs and lows.

Carb cycling offers a refreshing change. It's not about deprivation or extremes but finding balance—nourishing your body with the right nutrients at the right times. Whether you're here to shed stubborn pounds, enhance your workouts, or simply feel more energized throughout your day, this book will guide you through the principles and practices of carb cycling in a practical and sustainable way.

Throughout these pages, you'll discover how to tailor your carb intake to your lifestyle, leverage high-carb days for energy, navigate low-carb days for fat loss, and enjoy moderate-carb days for flexibility. Along the way, we'll address common challenges, celebrate your victories, and provide you with the tools you need to succeed.

So, if you're ready to embark on a journey that's not just about reaching your goals but also about embracing a healthier, more balanced approach to eating, let's dive in together.

- **What is Carb Cycling?**

Carb cycling is a dietary approach that involves alternating between high-carbohydrate days and low-carbohydrate days within a structured eating plan. The concept behind carb cycling is to strategically vary your carbohydrate intake based on your daily activity levels, fitness goals, and metabolic needs. This approach is often used by athletes, bodybuilders, and individuals seeking to optimize fat loss while preserving muscle mass.

Key Principles of Carb Cycling:

1. High-Carb Days:
   - On high-carb days, you consume a higher percentage of your calories from carbohydrates. This is typically aligned with days when you have intense physical activity or workouts planned. The increased carb intake helps replenish glycogen stores in your muscles and liver, providing energy for performance and promoting muscle recovery.

2. Low-Carb Days:
   - Low-carb days involve reducing your carbohydrate intake significantly, often to less than 20-30% of your total daily calories. These days are usually scheduled on rest days or days with lighter physical activity. By reducing carbs, your body is encouraged to burn stored fat for fuel, which can support fat loss goals.

3. Moderate-Carb Days:
   - Moderate-carb days fall between high and low-carb days in terms of carbohydrate intake. These days can provide a balance, supporting moderate physical activity or recovery days without drastically increasing or reducing carb intake.

Benefits of Carb Cycling:

- Improved Fat Loss: By cycling carbohydrates, you can optimize fat burning on low-carb days while still supporting muscle growth and recovery on high-carb days.

- Enhanced Muscle Retention: High-carb days help maintain muscle glycogen levels, which is crucial for muscle recovery and performance during workouts.

- Metabolic Flexibility: Carb cycling can improve your body's ability to switch between burning carbs and fats for fuel, enhancing overall metabolic efficiency.

- Sustainability: Unlike strict low-carb diets, carb cycling offers flexibility and can be easier to maintain long-term, reducing feelings of deprivation and monotony.

 Who Can Benefit from Carb Cycling:

- Athletes and Fitness Enthusiasts: Those looking to optimize performance and recovery while managing body composition.

- Weight Loss Seekers: Individuals aiming to lose body fat while preserving lean muscle mass.

- Metabolic Adaptation: People seeking to improve insulin sensitivity and overall metabolic health.

Carb cycling is not a one-size-fits-all approach, and its effectiveness may vary based on individual goals, body composition, and lifestyle. Adjustments to carb intake should be personalized based on individual needs and responses to ensure optimal results.

- Key Benefits

1. Optimized Fat Loss: By alternating between high-carb and low-carb days, carb cycling can enhance fat burning while preserving lean muscle mass. Low-carb days promote fat utilization for energy, especially during periods of rest or light activity, while high-carb days replenish glycogen stores and support intense workouts.

2. Preservation of Muscle Mass: High-carb days help maintain muscle glycogen levels, which is essential for muscle recovery and performance during workouts. This can prevent muscle breakdown that may occur with prolonged calorie restriction or very low-carb diets.

3. Enhanced Energy Levels: High-carb days provide a boost in energy, making it easier to perform well during workouts or physically demanding activities. Low-carb days encourage the body to become more efficient at using stored fat for fuel, which can also support sustained energy levels.

4. Improved Hormonal Balance: Carb cycling can help regulate hormones involved in metabolism and energy balance, such as insulin and leptin. This can lead to better appetite control, reduced cravings, and improved overall hormonal health.

5. Flexibility and Sustainability: Unlike strict low-carb diets, carb cycling offers flexibility in food choices and can be easier to maintain long-term. It allows for enjoyment of a variety of foods while still supporting health and fitness goals.

6. Metabolic Adaptation: Cycling between different carb intake levels can improve metabolic flexibility, helping the body become more efficient at using both carbs and fats for energy. This adaptation can enhance overall metabolic health and insulin sensitivity.

7. Personalization: Carb cycling can be tailored to individual needs, goals, and preferences. Whether your focus is on weight loss, muscle gain, or athletic performance, carb cycling can be adjusted to suit different activity levels and lifestyles.

Overall, carb cycling is a versatile dietary approach that can benefit individuals looking to optimize body composition, improve performance, and maintain overall health and well-being.

Chapter 1: The Basics

- Low, High, and Moderate Carb Days

Carb cycling revolves around the concept of strategically alternating between low, high, and moderate carbohydrate intake days to achieve specific health and fitness goals. Understanding the basics of each type of carb day is crucial for implementing this dietary strategy effectively.

Low-Carb Days

Low-carb days involve consuming a reduced amount of carbohydrates compared to your typical intake. The goal is to minimize insulin spikes and encourage the body to rely more on stored fat for energy. Typically, on low-carb days, carbohydrates may constitute around 10-20% of your total daily caloric intake. These days are often scheduled on rest days or days with minimal physical activity. By limiting carbs, your body enters a state of ketosis or fat adaptation, where it becomes efficient at burning fat for fuel. This can promote weight loss and improve metabolic flexibility over time.

High-Carb Days

High-carb days are characterized by consuming a higher proportion of carbohydrates, usually around 50-60% of your total daily caloric intake. These days are strategically planned around intense workouts or days when your energy demands are higher. The primary purpose of high-carb days is to replenish muscle glycogen stores and support optimal performance during training sessions. Carbohydrates are essential for providing immediate energy and promoting recovery by reducing muscle breakdown. High-carb days can help sustain muscle mass and improve overall workout quality, making them crucial for athletes and fitness enthusiasts.

Moderate-Carb Days

Moderate-carb days fall between low and high-carb days in terms of carbohydrate intake, typically constituting about 30-40% of your total daily caloric intake. These days offer a balanced approach, providing enough carbs to support moderate physical activity or recovery without the substantial glycogen replenishment seen on high-carb days. Moderate-carb days can enhance metabolic flexibility, allowing your body to efficiently switch between using carbohydrates and fats for fuel depending on activity levels.

Implementing Carb Cycling

Successfully implementing carb cycling involves understanding your individual energy needs, activity levels, and goals. Tailor your carb intake on different days based on your workout schedule, with high-carb days aligning with intense exercise sessions and low-carb days scheduled on rest days or light activity days. The goal is to optimize nutrient timing to support performance, enhance fat loss, and maintain muscle mass effectively.

By mastering the basics of low, high, and moderate carb days, you lay the foundation for a structured and effective carb cycling regimen that can adapt to your lifestyle and fitness goals over time. This approach not only enhances physical performance but also supports long-term metabolic health and overall well-being.

- Setting Goals

Setting clear and achievable goals is essential when embarking on a carb cycling journey. Here's how you can effectively set goals for your carb cycling plan:

Setting Goals for Carb Cycling

1. Define Your Objectives:
   - Start by identifying what you aim to achieve through carb cycling. Whether your goal is weight loss, muscle gain, improved athletic performance, or better overall health, clearly define your primary objectives. Having specific goals helps you stay focused and motivated throughout your journey.

2. Be Specific and Measurable:
   - Make your goals specific and measurable to track your progress effectively. For instance, instead of saying "I want to lose weight," specify how much weight you aim to lose within a certain timeframe, such as "I want to lose 10 pounds in the next 8 weeks."

3. Set Realistic Targets:
   - Ensure your goals are realistic and attainable based on your current fitness level, lifestyle, and commitment to the carb cycling plan. Unrealistic goals can lead to frustration and demotivation. Consider consulting with a nutritionist or fitness coach to help you set realistic targets.

4. Consider Timeframes:
   - Establish a timeline for achieving your goals. Short-term goals (e.g., weekly or monthly) can help you stay on track and celebrate small victories along the way. Long-term goals provide a broader perspective and help maintain momentum over time.

5. Break Down Goals into Steps:
   - Break down larger goals into smaller, actionable steps. This makes your goals more manageable and allows you to focus on making consistent progress. For example, if your goal is to improve athletic performance, your steps may include

setting training schedules, monitoring nutrition closely on high-performance days, and adjusting carb intake accordingly.

6. Account for Challenges:
   - Anticipate potential obstacles or challenges that may hinder your progress. Develop strategies to overcome these challenges, such as meal planning, managing cravings, or adjusting your carb cycling schedule as needed.

7. Monitor and Adjust:
   - Regularly monitor your progress towards your goals. Track measurements, changes in weight or body composition, performance improvements in workouts, and overall energy levels. Use this feedback to adjust your carb cycling plan as necessary to optimize results.

8. Stay Motivated:
   - Stay motivated by focusing on the benefits of achieving your goals. Celebrate milestones, reward yourself for progress, and surround yourself with support from friends, family, or online communities following similar journeys.

Example Goal Setting:
   - Example Goal: "I want to lose 10 pounds in the next 8 weeks by following a carb cycling plan."
   - Specific Action Steps:
     - Plan and prepare meals according to carb cycling guidelines.
       - Exercise at least 4 times a week, aligning high-carb days with intense workouts.
     - Track progress weekly using measurements and photos.
     - Adjust carb intake based on energy levels and workout performance.

By setting clear, specific, and realistic goals for your carb cycling journey, you can effectively tailor your approach to meet your individual needs and achieve sustainable results over time.

Chapter 2: High-Carb Days Recipes

High Carb Breakfast

1. Banana Oat Pancakes

Ingredients:
- 1 cup rolled oats
- 1 ripe banana
- 1 cup milk (dairy or non-dairy)
- 1 egg
- 1 tsp baking powder
- 1 tsp vanilla extract
- 1 tbsp honey or maple syrup
- Pinch of salt
- Cooking spray or butter for the pan

Instructions:
1. Blend the oats in a blender until they form a fine flour.
2. Add the banana, milk, egg, baking powder, vanilla extract, honey, and salt to the blender. Blend until smooth.
3. Heat a non-stick skillet over medium heat and lightly coat with cooking spray or butter.
4. Pour 1/4 cup of batter onto the skillet for each pancake. Cook until bubbles form on the surface, then flip and cook until golden brown on the other side.
5. Serve with additional banana slices and a drizzle of honey or maple syrup.

2. Sweet Potato Breakfast Hash

Ingredients:
- 2 medium sweet potatoes, peeled and diced
- 1 red bell pepper, diced
- 1 green bell pepper, diced
- 1 small onion, diced
- 2 cloves garlic, minced

- 2 tbsp olive oil
- 1 tsp paprika
- 1/2 tsp cumin
- Salt and pepper to taste
- 4 eggs
- Fresh parsley for garnish

Instructions:
1. Heat olive oil in a large skillet over medium heat.
2. Add the sweet potatoes, bell peppers, and onion. Cook until the vegetables are tender, about 10-15 minutes.
3. Add the garlic, paprika, cumin, salt, and pepper. Cook for another 2-3 minutes.
4. Create four small wells in the hash and crack an egg into each well.
5. Cover the skillet and cook until the eggs are set to your liking, about 5-7 minutes.
6. Garnish with fresh parsley and serve.

3. Apple Cinnamon Overnight Oats

Ingredients:
- 1 cup rolled oats
- 1 cup milk (dairy or non-dairy)
- 1/2 cup unsweetened applesauce
- 1/2 tsp ground cinnamon
- 1 tbsp chia seeds
- 1 tbsp maple syrup or honey
- 1 apple, diced
- Nuts or seeds for topping (optional)

Instructions:
1. In a jar or container, combine the oats, milk, applesauce, cinnamon, chia seeds, and maple syrup. Stir well.
2. Cover and refrigerate overnight.
3. In the morning, top with diced apple and nuts or seeds if desired.

4. Quinoa Breakfast Bowl

Ingredients:
- 1 cup cooked quinoa
- 1/2 cup Greek yogurt
- 1 banana, sliced
- 1/2 cup mixed berries
- 1 tbsp honey or maple syrup
- 1 tbsp chia seeds
- 1 tbsp chopped nuts

Instructions:
1. In a bowl, combine the cooked quinoa and Greek yogurt.
2. Top with banana slices, mixed berries, honey, chia seeds, and chopped nuts.
3. Serve immediately.

5. Blueberry Muffin Smoothie

Ingredients:
- 1 cup frozen blueberries
- 1/2 cup rolled oats
- 1 banana
- 1 cup milk (dairy or non-dairy)
- 1/2 cup Greek yogurt
- 1 tsp vanilla extract
- 1 tbsp honey or maple syrup

Instructions:
1. Place all ingredients in a blender and blend until smooth.
2. Pour into a glass and enjoy.

6. Strawberry Banana Smoothie Bowl

Ingredients:
- 1 cup frozen strawberries

- 1 frozen banana
- 1/2 cup rolled oats
- 1/2 cup Greek yogurt
- 1/2 cup milk (dairy or non-dairy)
- 1 tbsp honey or maple syrup
- Toppings: fresh fruit, granola, chia seeds, coconut flakes

Instructions:
1. Blend the frozen strawberries, banana, oats, Greek yogurt, milk, and honey until smooth.
2. Pour into a bowl and top with fresh fruit, granola, chia seeds, and coconut flakes.

7. Peanut Butter Banana Toast

Ingredients:
- 2 slices whole grain bread
- 2 tbsp peanut butter
- 1 banana, sliced
- 1 tsp honey
- 1/2 tsp cinnamon

Instructions:
1. Toast the bread slices.
2. Spread peanut butter on each slice.
3. Top with banana slices.
4. Drizzle with honey and sprinkle with cinnamon.

8. Maple Walnut Baked Oatmeal

Ingredients:
- 2 cups rolled oats
- 1/2 cup chopped walnuts
- 1 tsp baking powder
- 1/2 tsp ground cinnamon
- 1/4 tsp salt

- 2 cups milk (dairy or non-dairy)
- 1/4 cup maple syrup
- 1 large egg
- 2 tbsp melted butter or coconut oil
- 1 tsp vanilla extract

Instructions:
1. Preheat the oven to 375°F (190°C).
2. In a large bowl, mix the oats, walnuts, baking powder, cinnamon, and salt.
3. In another bowl, whisk together the milk, maple syrup, egg, melted butter, and vanilla extract.
4. Pour the wet ingredients into the dry ingredients and mix well.
5. Pour the mixture into a greased baking dish.
6. Bake for 35-40 minutes, until the top is golden brown and the oatmeal is set.
7. Serve warm, drizzled with additional maple syrup if desired.

9. Mango Chia Pudding

Ingredients:
- 1 cup coconut milk
- 1/4 cup chia seeds
- 1 ripe mango, peeled and diced
- 1 tbsp honey or maple syrup
- 1/2 tsp vanilla extract

Instructions:
1. In a bowl, mix the coconut milk, chia seeds, honey, and vanilla extract.
2. Let the mixture sit for about 5 minutes, then stir again to prevent clumping.
3. Cover and refrigerate for at least 4 hours, or overnight.
4. Before serving, top with diced mango.

10. Sweet Potato Smoothie

Ingredients:
- 1 cup cooked sweet potato, cooled

- 1 banana
- 1/2 cup Greek yogurt
- 1 cup milk (dairy or non-dairy)
- 1 tbsp honey or maple syrup
- 1/2 tsp ground cinnamon
- 1/4 tsp ground nutmeg

Instructions:
1. Place all ingredients in a blender and blend until smooth.
2. Pour into a glass and enjoy.

High Carb Lunch

1. Chicken Burrito Bowl

Ingredients:
- 1 cup cooked brown rice
- 1 chicken breast, cooked and shredded
- 1/2 cup black beans, drained and rinsed
- 1/2 cup corn kernels
- 1/2 avocado, diced
- 1/2 cup cherry tomatoes, halved
- 1/4 cup shredded cheddar cheese
- 2 tbsp salsa
- 1 tbsp sour cream
- 1 lime, cut into wedges
- Fresh cilantro for garnish

Instructions:
1. In a bowl, layer the brown rice, shredded chicken, black beans, corn, avocado, cherry tomatoes, and cheddar cheese.
2. Top with salsa and sour cream.
3. Garnish with fresh cilantro and lime wedges.
4. Serve immediately.

2. Sweet Potato and Black Bean Tacos

Ingredients:
- 2 medium sweet potatoes, peeled and diced
- 1 can black beans, drained and rinsed
- 1 tbsp olive oil
- 1 tsp cumin
- 1/2 tsp chili powder
- Salt and pepper to taste
- 8 small corn tortillas
- 1/2 cup shredded lettuce

- 1/4 cup diced red onion
- 1/2 cup diced tomatoes
- 1/4 cup crumbled feta cheese
- Fresh cilantro for garnish
- Lime wedges

Instructions:
1. Preheat oven to 400°F (200°C).
2. Toss the diced sweet potatoes with olive oil, cumin, chili powder, salt, and pepper.
3. Spread on a baking sheet and roast for 20-25 minutes, until tender.
4. Warm the tortillas in a dry skillet over medium heat.
5. Fill each tortilla with roasted sweet potatoes, black beans, lettuce, red onion, tomatoes, and feta cheese.
6. Garnish with fresh cilantro and lime wedges.
7. Serve immediately.

3. Vegetable Stir-Fry with Rice Noodles

Ingredients:
- 8 oz rice noodles
- 1 tbsp vegetable oil
- 1 red bell pepper, sliced
- 1 yellow bell pepper, sliced
- 1 cup snap peas
- 1 cup broccoli florets
- 1 carrot, julienned
- 2 cloves garlic, minced
- 1 tbsp soy sauce
- 1 tbsp hoisin sauce
- 1 tsp sesame oil
- 1 tbsp sesame seeds
- Green onions for garnish

Instructions:
1. Cook the rice noodles according to package instructions. Drain and set aside.
2. Heat vegetable oil in a large skillet or wok over medium-high heat.
3. Add the bell peppers, snap peas, broccoli, and carrot. Stir-fry for 5-7 minutes, until the vegetables are tender-crisp.
4. Add the garlic and stir-fry for another minute.
5. Stir in the cooked rice noodles, soy sauce, hoisin sauce, and sesame oil. Toss to combine.
6. Garnish with sesame seeds and green onions.
7. Serve immediately.

4. Quinoa and Chickpea Salad

Ingredients:
- 1 cup cooked quinoa
- 1 can chickpeas, drained and rinsed
- 1/2 cucumber, diced
- 1/2 cup cherry tomatoes, halved
- 1/4 red onion, diced
- 1/4 cup crumbled feta cheese
- 2 tbsp olive oil
- 1 tbsp lemon juice
- 1 tsp dried oregano
- Salt and pepper to taste
- Fresh parsley for garnish

Instructions:
1. In a large bowl, combine the cooked quinoa, chickpeas, cucumber, cherry tomatoes, red onion, and feta cheese.
2. In a small bowl, whisk together the olive oil, lemon juice, oregano, salt, and pepper.
3. Pour the dressing over the salad and toss to combine.
4. Garnish with fresh parsley.
5. Serve chilled or at room temperature.

5. Pasta Primavera

Ingredients:
- 8 oz whole wheat pasta
- 1 tbsp olive oil
- 1 zucchini, sliced
- 1 yellow squash, sliced
- 1 red bell pepper, sliced
- 1 cup cherry tomatoes, halved
- 2 cloves garlic, minced
- 1/2 cup grated Parmesan cheese
- 1/4 cup fresh basil, chopped
- Salt and pepper to taste

Instructions:
1. Cook the pasta according to package instructions. Drain and set aside.
2. Heat olive oil in a large skillet over medium heat.
3. Add the zucchini, yellow squash, and red bell pepper. Cook for 5-7 minutes, until the vegetables are tender.
4. Add the cherry tomatoes and garlic. Cook for another 2-3 minutes.
5. Add the cooked pasta to the skillet and toss to combine.
6. Stir in the Parmesan cheese, fresh basil, salt, and pepper.
7. Serve immediately.

6. Lentil and Brown Rice Soup

Ingredients:
- 1 cup lentils, rinsed
- 1/2 cup brown rice
- 1 tbsp olive oil
- 1 onion, diced
- 2 carrots, diced
- 2 celery stalks, diced
- 2 cloves garlic, minced
- 6 cups vegetable broth

- 1 can diced tomatoes
- 1 tsp cumin
- 1/2 tsp thyme
- Salt and pepper to taste
- Fresh parsley for garnish

Instructions:
1. In a large pot, heat the olive oil over medium heat.
2. Add the onion, carrots, and celery. Cook until the vegetables are softened, about 5-7 minutes.
3. Add the garlic and cook for another minute.
4. Stir in the lentils, brown rice, vegetable broth, diced tomatoes, cumin, thyme, salt, and pepper.
5. Bring to a boil, then reduce the heat and simmer for 30-35 minutes, until the lentils and rice are tender.
6. Garnish with fresh parsley.
7. Serve hot.

7. Falafel Wraps

Ingredients:
- 1 can chickpeas, drained and rinsed
- 1 small onion, diced
- 2 cloves garlic, minced
- 1/4 cup fresh parsley
- 1/4 cup fresh cilantro
- 1 tsp cumin
- 1/2 tsp coriander
- Salt and pepper to taste
- 3 tbsp flour
- 2 tbsp olive oil
- 4 whole wheat tortillas
- 1/2 cup hummus
- 1 cup shredded lettuce
- 1/2 cup diced tomatoes

- 1/4 cup sliced red onion

Instructions:
1. In a food processor, combine the chickpeas, onion, garlic, parsley, cilantro, cumin, coriander, salt, and pepper. Pulse until combined but still slightly chunky.
2. Transfer the mixture to a bowl and stir in the flour.
3. Form the mixture into small patties.
4. Heat olive oil in a large skillet over medium heat. Cook the patties for 3-4 minutes on each side, until golden brown.
5. Warm the tortillas in a dry skillet over medium heat.
6. Spread hummus on each tortilla, then top with falafel patties, lettuce, tomatoes, and red onion.
7. Wrap tightly and serve.

8. Thai Peanut Noodles

Ingredients:
- 8 oz rice noodles
- 1/4 cup peanut butter
- 2 tbsp soy sauce
- 1 tbsp rice vinegar
- 1 tbsp honey
- 1 tbsp lime juice
- 1 tsp sesame oil
- 1/2 tsp crushed red pepper flakes
- 1 red bell pepper, sliced
- 1 carrot, julienned
- 1/2 cup shredded purple cabbage
- 1/4 cup chopped peanuts
- Fresh cilantro for garnish

Instructions:
1. Cook the rice noodles according to package instructions. Drain and set aside.
2. In a small bowl, whisk together the peanut butter, soy sauce, rice vinegar, honey, lime juice, sesame oil, and red pepper flakes.

3. In a large bowl, combine the cooked noodles, bell pepper, carrot, and cabbage.
4. Pour the peanut sauce over the noodles and toss to combine.
5. Garnish with chopped peanuts and fresh cilantro.
6. Serve immediately.

 9. Butternut Squash Risotto

Ingredients:
- 1 cup Arborio rice
- 4 cups vegetable broth
- 1 small butternut squash, peeled and diced
- 1 small onion, diced
- 2 cloves garlic, minced
- 1/2 cup dry white wine
- 1/4 cup grated Parmesan cheese
- 2 tbsp olive oil
- Salt and pepper to taste
- Fresh sage for garnish

Instructions:
1. Heat the vegetable broth in a saucepan over low heat.
2. In a large skillet, heat the olive oil over medium heat. Add the butternut squash and cook until tender, about 10-12 minutes. Remove and set aside.
3. In the same skillet, add the onion and cook until translucent, about 5 minutes.
4. Add the garlic and cook for another minute.
5. Stir in the Arborio rice and cook for 2-3 minutes until slightly toasted.
6. Add the white wine and cook until absorbed.
7. Add the vegetable broth, one ladle at a time, stirring frequently and allowing each addition to be absorbed before adding the nextaddition. Continue this process until the rice is creamy and cooked through, about 18-20 minutes.
8. Stir in the cooked butternut squash and Parmesan cheese. Season with salt and pepper to taste.
9. Garnish with fresh sage.
10. Serve immediately.

10. Mediterranean Grain Bowl

Ingredients:
- 1 cup cooked farro or quinoa
- 1/2 cup cherry tomatoes, halved
- 1/2 cucumber, diced
- 1/4 red onion, thinly sliced
- 1/4 cup Kalamata olives, pitted and halved
- 1/4 cup crumbled feta cheese
- 2 tbsp olive oil
- 1 tbsp lemon juice
- 1 tsp dried oregano
- Salt and pepper to taste
- Fresh parsley for garnish

Instructions:
1. In a large bowl, combine the cooked farro or quinoa, cherry tomatoes, cucumber, red onion, olives, and feta cheese.
2. In a small bowl, whisk together the olive oil, lemon juice, oregano, salt, and pepper.
3. Pour the dressing over the grain bowl and toss to combine.
4. Garnish with fresh parsley.
5. Serve chilled or at room temperature.

High Carb Dinner

1. Vegetable Lasagna

Ingredients:
- 9 lasagna noodles
- 2 cups ricotta cheese
- 1 egg
- 2 cups shredded mozzarella cheese
- 1/2 cup grated Parmesan cheese
- 2 cups marinara sauce
- 1 zucchini, sliced
- 1 yellow squash, sliced
- 1 cup spinach
- 1 red bell pepper, sliced
- 1 tbsp olive oil
- Salt and pepper to taste
- Fresh basil for garnish

Instructions:
1. Preheat the oven to 375°F (190°C).
2. Cook lasagna noodles according to package instructions. Drain and set aside.
3. In a large skillet, heat olive oil over medium heat. Add zucchini, yellow squash, and red bell pepper. Cook until tender, about 5-7 minutes. Add spinach and cook until wilted. Season with salt and pepper.
4. In a bowl, mix ricotta cheese, egg, and Parmesan cheese.
5. Spread a thin layer of marinara sauce in a 9x13 inch baking dish. Place three lasagna noodles on top.
6. Spread 1/3 of the ricotta mixture over the noodles, followed by 1/3 of the vegetable mixture, and 1/3 of the mozzarella cheese. Repeat layers twice.
7. Finish with a layer of marinara sauce and the remaining mozzarella cheese.
8. Cover with foil and bake for 25 minutes. Remove foil and bake for another 15 minutes, until cheese is bubbly and golden.
9. Garnish with fresh basil and serve.

2. Chickpea and Spinach Curry

Ingredients:
- 1 tbsp olive oil
- 1 onion, diced
- 2 cloves garlic, minced
- 1 tbsp ginger, grated
- 1 tbsp curry powder
- 1 tsp cumin
- 1/2 tsp turmeric
- 1 can diced tomatoes
- 1 can coconut milk
- 2 cans chickpeas, drained and rinsed
- 4 cups fresh spinach
- Salt and pepper to taste
- Fresh cilantro for garnish
- Cooked rice, for serving

Instructions:
1. Heat olive oil in a large pot over medium heat. Add onion and cook until softened, about 5 minutes.
2. Add garlic and ginger, cook for another minute.
3. Stir in curry powder, cumin, and turmeric. Cook for 1-2 minutes until fragrant.
4. Add diced tomatoes and coconut milk. Bring to a simmer.
5. Add chickpeas and spinach. Cook until spinach is wilted and chickpeas are heated through, about 5-7 minutes.
6. Season with salt and pepper.
7. Garnish with fresh cilantro and serve over cooked rice.

3. Sweet Potato and Black Bean Enchiladas

Ingredients:
- 2 large sweet potatoes, peeled and diced
- 1 tbsp olive oil
- 1 can black beans, drained and rinsed

- 1 cup corn kernels
- 2 cups enchilada sauce
- 8 whole wheat tortillas
- 1 cup shredded cheddar cheese
- 1/2 cup diced red onion
- 1/4 cup chopped fresh cilantro
- Salt and pepper to taste

Instructions:
1. Preheat oven to 375°F (190°C).
2. Toss diced sweet potatoes with olive oil, salt, and pepper. Spread on a baking sheet and roast for 20-25 minutes, until tender.
3. In a large bowl, combine roasted sweet potatoes, black beans, corn, and 1 cup of enchilada sauce.
4. Spoon mixture into tortillas, roll up, and place seam-side down in a baking dish.
5. Pour remaining enchilada sauce over the top and sprinkle with cheddar cheese.
6. Bake for 20-25 minutes, until cheese is melted and bubbly.
7. Garnish with diced red onion and fresh cilantro.
8. Serve immediately.

4. Spaghetti Carbonara

Ingredients:
- 12 oz spaghetti
- 4 slices bacon, chopped
- 3 cloves garlic, minced
- 2 large eggs
- 1 cup grated Parmesan cheese
- 1/2 cup heavy cream
- Salt and pepper to taste
- Fresh parsley for garnish

Instructions:
1. Cook spaghetti according to package instructions. Drain, reserving 1 cup of pasta water.

2. In a large skillet, cook bacon over medium heat until crispy. Remove and set aside, leaving the drippings in the skillet.

3. Add garlic to the skillet and cook for 1-2 minutes until fragrant.

4. In a bowl, whisk together eggs, Parmesan cheese, and heavy cream.

5. Return the spaghetti to the skillet, tossing to coat in bacon drippings. Remove from heat.

6. Quickly stir in the egg mixture, tossing to coat the pasta. Add reserved pasta water as needed to reach desired consistency.

7. Stir in cooked bacon and season with salt and pepper.

8. Garnish with fresh parsley and serve immediately.

5. Vegetable Paella

Ingredients:
- 1 tbsp olive oil
- 1 onion, diced
- 2 cloves garlic, minced
- 1 red bell pepper, sliced
- 1 yellow bell pepper, sliced
- 1 cup green beans, trimmed
- 1 cup cherry tomatoes, halved
- 1 1/2 cups Arborio rice
- 4 cups vegetable broth
- 1 tsp saffron threads
- 1 tsp smoked paprika
- Salt and pepper to taste
- Fresh lemon wedges and parsley for garnish

Instructions:

1. In a large pan, heat olive oil over medium heat. Add onion and garlic, cook until softened, about 5 minutes.

2. Add red and yellow bell peppers, green beans, and cherry tomatoes. Cook for another 5 minutes.

3. Stir in Arborio rice, saffron, smoked paprika, salt, and pepper.

4. Gradually add vegetable broth, stirring frequently, until the rice is tender and the liquid is absorbed, about 20-25 minutes.
5. Garnish with fresh lemon wedges and parsley.
6. Serve immediately.

6. Lemon Herb Risotto

Ingredients:
- 1 cup Arborio rice
- 4 cups vegetable broth
- 1 small onion, diced
- 2 cloves garlic, minced
- 1/2 cup dry white wine
- 1 lemon, zested and juiced
- 1/4 cup grated Parmesan cheese
- 2 tbsp butter
- 2 tbsp fresh parsley, chopped
- Salt and pepper to taste

Instructions:
1. Heat the vegetable broth in a saucepan over low heat.
2. In a large skillet, melt butter over medium heat. Add onion and cook until translucent, about 5 minutes.
3. Add garlic and cook for another minute.
4. Stir in Arborio rice and cook for 2-3 minutes until slightly toasted.
5. Add white wine and cook until absorbed.
6. Gradually add vegetable broth, one ladle at a time, stirring frequently and allowing each addition to be absorbed before adding the next.
7. Once the rice is creamy and cooked through, stir in lemon zest, lemon juice, Parmesan cheese, salt, and pepper.
8. Garnish with fresh parsley.
9. Serve immediately.

7. Mushroom Stroganoff

Ingredients:
- 1 tbsp olive oil
- 1 onion, diced
- 3 cloves garlic, minced
- 2 cups mushrooms, sliced
- 1 tbsp flour
- 1 cup vegetable broth
- 1/2 cup sour cream
- 1 tbsp Dijon mustard
- 2 cups cooked egg noodles
- Salt and pepper to taste
- Fresh parsley for garnish

Instructions:
1. Heat olive oil in a large skillet over medium heat. Add onion and cook until softened, about 5 minutes.
2. Add garlic and mushrooms, cook until mushrooms are tender and browned, about 5-7 minutes.
3. Sprinkle flour over the mushrooms and stir to combine.
4. Gradually stir in vegetable broth and bring to a simmer. Cook until thickened, about 3-5 minutes.
5. Stir in sour cream and Dijon mustard. Season with salt and pepper.
6. Add cooked egg noodles and toss to coat.
7. Garnish with fresh parsley.
8. Serve immediately.

8. Baked Ziti

Ingredients:
- 12 oz ziti pasta
- 1 tbsp olive oil
- 1 onion, diced
- 3 cloves garlic, minced

- 1 lb ground beef or turkey
- 4 cups marinara sauce
- 1 cup ricotta cheese
- 2 cups shredded mozzarella cheese
- 1/2 cup grated Parmesan cheese
- Salt and pepper to taste
- Fresh basil for garnish

Instructions:
1. Preheat oven to 375°F (190°C).
2. Cook ziti pasta according to package instructions. Drain and set aside.
3. In a large skillet, heat olive oil over medium heat. Add onion and garlic, cook until softened, about 5 minutes.
4. Add ground beef or turkey and cook until browned. Drain any excess fat.
5. Stir in marinara sauce and simmer for 10 minutes. Season with salt and pepper.
6. In a large bowl, combine cooked ziti pasta, ricotta cheese, and 1 cup of mozzarella cheese.
7. Spread half of the pasta mixture in a 9x13 inch baking dish. Top with half of the meat sauce. Repeatwith the remaining pasta mixture and meat sauce. Sprinkle the remaining 1 cup of mozzarella cheese and Parmesan cheese on top.
8. Cover with foil and bake for 20 minutes. Remove foil and bake for an additional 10-15 minutes, until cheese is melted and bubbly.
9. Garnish with fresh basil.
10. Serve immediately.

9. Stuffed Peppers

Ingredients:
- 4 large bell peppers (any color)
- 1 cup quinoa, cooked
- 1 can black beans, drained and rinsed
- 1 cup corn kernels
- 1 cup diced tomatoes
- 1/2 cup diced red onion
- 1 tsp cumin

- 1 tsp chili powder
- Salt and pepper to taste
- 1 cup shredded cheddar cheese
- Fresh cilantro for garnish

Instructions:
1. Preheat oven to 375°F (190°C).
2. Cut the tops off the bell peppers and remove seeds and membranes. Place the peppers in a baking dish.
3. In a large bowl, combine cooked quinoa, black beans, corn, diced tomatoes, red onion, cumin, chili powder, salt, and pepper.
4. Spoon the mixture into the bell peppers, packing it down gently.
5. Sprinkle shredded cheddar cheese on top of each stuffed pepper.
6. Cover with foil and bake for 25 minutes. Remove foil and bake for an additional 10-15 minutes, until cheese is melted and peppers are tender.
7. Garnish with fresh cilantro.
8. Serve immediately.

10. Lentil Shepherd's Pie

Ingredients:
- 1 tbsp olive oil
- 1 onion, diced
- 2 cloves garlic, minced
- 2 carrots, diced
- 2 celery stalks, diced
- 1 cup green or brown lentils, rinsed
- 2 cups vegetable broth
- 1 cup frozen peas
- 1 tbsp tomato paste
- 1 tsp thyme
- 1 tsp rosemary
- Salt and pepper to taste
- 4 cups mashed potatoes
- Fresh parsley for garnish

Instructions:
1. Preheat oven to 400°F (200°C).
2. In a large skillet, heat olive oil over medium heat. Add onion, garlic, carrots, and celery. Cook until vegetables are softened, about 5-7 minutes.
3. Add lentils, vegetable broth, tomato paste, thyme, rosemary, salt, and pepper. Bring to a boil, then reduce heat and simmer until lentils are tender and most of the liquid is absorbed, about 25-30 minutes.
4. Stir in frozen peas and cook for another 5 minutes.
5. Transfer the lentil mixture to a baking dish and spread evenly.
6. Spoon mashed potatoes over the top, spreading them out to cover the lentil mixture completely.
7. Bake for 20-25 minutes, until the top is golden brown.
8. Garnish with fresh parsley.
9. Serve immediately.

High Carb Snacks

1. Banana Peanut Butter Toast

Ingredients:
- 1 slice whole grain bread
- 1 tbsp peanut butter
- 1 banana, sliced
- 1 tsp honey (optional)
- 1/2 tsp chia seeds (optional)

Instructions:
1. Toast the bread until golden brown.
2. Spread peanut butter evenly over the toast.
3. Arrange banana slices on top.
4. Drizzle with honey and sprinkle with chia seeds if desired.

2. Greek Yogurt with Granola and Berries

Ingredients:
- 1 cup Greek yogurt
- 1/2 cup granola
- 1/2 cup mixed berries (strawberries, blueberries, raspberries)
- 1 tbsp honey

Instructions:
1. Scoop the Greek yogurt into a bowl.
2. Top with granola and mixed berries.
3. Drizzle with honey before serving.

3. Hummus and Pita Chips

Ingredients:
- 1 cup hummus
- 1 pita bread, cut into chips

- 1 tbsp olive oil
- Salt to taste

Instructions:
1. Preheat the oven to 375°F (190°C).
2. Brush pita chips with olive oil and sprinkle with salt.
3. Bake for 10-12 minutes until crispy.
4. Serve with hummus.

4. Trail Mix

Ingredients:
- 1 cup mixed nuts (almonds, cashews, walnuts)
- 1/2 cup dried fruit (raisins, cranberries, apricots)
- 1/4 cup dark chocolate chips
- 1/4 cup sunflower seeds

Instructions:
1. Mix all ingredients in a bowl.
2. Store in an airtight container.

5. Fruit Smoothie

Ingredients:
- 1 banana
- 1/2 cup strawberries
- 1/2 cup blueberries
- 1 cup almond milk
- 1 tbsp honey
- 1/2 cup Greek yogurt

Instructions:
1. Combine all ingredients in a blender.
2. Blend until smooth.
3. Pour into a glass and serve immediately.

6. Apple Slices with Almond Butter

Ingredients:
- 1 apple, sliced
- 2 tbsp almond butter
- 1 tbsp granola (optional)
- 1 tsp cinnamon (optional)

Instructions:
1. Arrange apple slices on a plate.
2. Spread almond butter on each slice.
3. Sprinkle with granola and cinnamon if desired.

7. Oatmeal with Honey and Berries

Ingredients:
- 1/2 cup rolled oats
- 1 cup water or milk
- 1 tbsp honey
- 1/2 cup mixed berries

Instructions:
1. Cook oats according to package instructions.
2. Stir in honey.
3. Top with mixed berries before serving.

8. Rice Cakes with Avocado and Tomato

Ingredients:
- 2 rice cakes
- 1 avocado, mashed
- 1 small tomato, sliced
- Salt and pepper to taste

Instructions:
1. Spread mashed avocado evenly over rice cakes.
2. Top with tomato slices.
3. Season with salt and pepper.

9. Sweet Potato Fries

Ingredients:
- 2 large sweet potatoes, cut into fries
- 2 tbsp olive oil
- 1/2 tsp paprika
- 1/2 tsp garlic powder
- Salt to taste

Instructions:
1. Preheat the oven to 425°F (220°C).
2. Toss sweet potato fries with olive oil, paprika, garlic powder, and salt.
3. Spread fries on a baking sheet in a single layer.
4. Bake for 20-25 minutes until crispy, flipping halfway through.

10. Chia Pudding with Fruit

Ingredients:
- 1/4 cup chia seeds
- 1 cup almond milk
- 1 tbsp honey
- 1/2 cup diced fruit (mango, berries, kiwi)

Instructions:
1. In a bowl, mix chia seeds, almond milk, and honey.
2. Stir well to combine.
3. Refrigerate for at least 4 hours or overnight.
4. Top with diced fruit before serving.

Chapter 3: Low-Carb Days Recipes

LOW carb Breakfast

1. Keto Avocado and Egg Breakfast Bowl

Ingredients:
- 1 ripe avocado
- 2 large eggs
- 1 tbsp olive oil
- Salt and pepper to taste
- Red pepper flakes (optional)
- Fresh cilantro for garnish

Instructions:
1. Halve the avocado and remove the pit. Scoop out a little of the flesh to make room for the egg.
2. Heat olive oil in a skillet over medium heat.
3. Crack the eggs into the skillet and cook until whites are set and yolks are cooked to your liking.
4. Place the eggs into the avocado halves.
5. Season with salt, pepper, and red pepper flakes if desired.
6. Garnish with fresh cilantro and serve immediately.

2. Low-Carb Veggie Omelette

Ingredients:
- 2 large eggs
- 1/4 cup diced bell peppers
- 1/4 cup diced onions
- 1/4 cup spinach, chopped
- 1/4 cup mushrooms, sliced
- 1/4 cup shredded cheese (optional)
- 1 tbsp butter
- Salt and pepper to taste

Instructions:

1. Beat the eggs in a bowl and season with salt and pepper.
2. Melt butter in a non-stick skillet over medium heat.
3. Add bell peppers, onions, spinach, and mushrooms. Cook until tender, about 5 minutes.
4. Pour the beaten eggs over the veggies.
5. Cook until the eggs are almost set, then sprinkle with cheese if using.
6. Fold the omelette in half and cook for another minute.
7. Serve immediately.

3. Greek Yogurt with Nuts and Berries

Ingredients:
- 1 cup Greek yogurt
- 1/4 cup mixed berries (strawberries, blueberries, raspberries)
- 2 tbsp chopped nuts (almonds, walnuts)
- 1 tsp chia seeds
- 1 tsp honey (optional)

Instructions:

1. Scoop the Greek yogurt into a bowl.
2. Top with mixed berries, chopped nuts, and chia seeds.
3. Drizzle with honey if desired.
4. Serve immediately.

4. Low-Carb Breakfast Muffins

Ingredients:
- 6 large eggs
- 1/2 cup diced bell peppers
- 1/2 cup diced onions
- 1/2 cup chopped spinach
- 1/2 cup shredded cheese (optional)
- Salt and pepper to taste
- Non-stick cooking spray

Instructions:
1. Preheat oven to 375°F (190°C).
2. In a bowl, beat the eggs and season with salt and pepper.
3. Stir in bell peppers, onions, spinach, and cheese if using.
4. Spray a muffin tin with non-stick cooking spray.
5. Pour the egg mixture into the muffin cups, filling each about 3/4 full.
6. Bake for 20-25 minutes, until the muffins are set and golden.
7. Serve warm.

5. Chia Seed Pudding

Ingredients:
- 1/4 cup chia seeds
- 1 cup unsweetened almond milk
- 1 tsp vanilla extract
- 1 tbsp sweetener of choice (optional)
- Fresh berries for topping

Instructions:
1. In a bowl, combine chia seeds, almond milk, vanilla extract, and sweetener if using.
2. Stir well to combine.
3. Cover and refrigerate for at least 4 hours, or overnight.
4. Stir again before serving and top with fresh berries.
5. Serve chilled.

6. Smoked Salmon and Avocado Salad

Ingredients:
- 1 avocado, sliced
- 4 oz smoked salmon
- 1 cup mixed greens
- 1 tbsp capers
- 1 tbsp olive oil
- 1 tbsp lemon juice

- Salt and pepper to taste

Instructions:
1. Arrange mixed greens on a plate.
2. Top with sliced avocado and smoked salmon.
3. Sprinkle with capers.
4. Drizzle with olive oil and lemon juice.
5. Season with salt and pepper.
6. Serve immediately.

 7. Cottage Cheese with Tomatoes and Cucumber

Ingredients:
- 1 cup cottage cheese
- 1/2 cup cherry tomatoes, halved
- 1/2 cucumber, diced
- 1 tbsp olive oil
- Salt and pepper to taste
- Fresh basil for garnish

Instructions:
1. Scoop the cottage cheese into a bowl.
2. Top with cherry tomatoes and cucumber.
3. Drizzle with olive oil.
4. Season with salt and pepper.
5. Garnish with fresh basil.
6. Serve immediately.

 8. Spinach and Feta Stuffed Mushrooms

Ingredients:
- 4 large portobello mushrooms
- 1 cup spinach, chopped
- 1/2 cup feta cheese, crumbled
- 1 tbsp olive oil

- 1 clove garlic, minced
- Salt and pepper to taste

Instructions:
1. Preheat oven to 375°F (190°C).
2. Remove stems from mushrooms and scoop out the gills.
3. In a skillet, heat olive oil over medium heat. Add garlic and spinach, cooking until spinach is wilted.
4. Stir in feta cheese and season with salt and pepper.
5. Stuff each mushroom cap with the spinach mixture.
6. Place the stuffed mushrooms on a baking sheet and bake for 15-20 minutes.
7. Serve warm.

9. Cauliflower Hash Browns

Ingredients:
- 2 cups grated cauliflower
- 1 egg
- 1/4 cup grated Parmesan cheese
- 1/4 cup almond flour
- 1/2 tsp garlic powder
- Salt and pepper to taste
- 2 tbsp olive oil

Instructions:
1. In a bowl, combine grated cauliflower, egg, Parmesan cheese, almond flour, garlic powder, salt, and pepper.
2. Heat olive oil in a skillet over medium heat.
3. Scoop about 1/4 cup of the cauliflower mixture and form it into a patty. Place in the skillet.
4. Cook for 3-4 minutes on each side, until golden brown and crispy.
5. Repeat with remaining mixture.
6. Serve warm.

10. Keto Pancakes

Ingredients:
- 1/2 cup almond flour
- 2 large eggs
- 1/4 cup cream cheese, softened
- 1/2 tsp baking powder
- 1 tsp vanilla extract
- Butter or coconut oil for cooking

Instructions:
1. In a blender, combine almond flour, eggs, cream cheese, baking powder, and vanilla extract. Blend until smooth.
2. Heat butter or coconut oil in a skillet over medium heat.
3. Pour 1/4 cup of batter into the skillet and cook until bubbles form on the surface, about 2-3 minutes. Flip and cook for another 1-2 minutes.
4. Repeat with remaining batter.
5. Serve warm with low-carb syrup or berries.

Low Carb Lunch

1. Zucchini Noodles with Pesto and Cherry Tomatoes

Ingredients:
- 2 medium zucchinis
- 1/2 cup cherry tomatoes, halved
- 1/4 cup pesto sauce
- 2 tbsp olive oil
- 1/4 cup grated Parmesan cheese
- Salt and pepper to taste

Instructions:
1. Spiralize the zucchinis to make zucchini noodles.
2. Heat olive oil in a large skillet over medium heat.
3. Add the zucchini noodles and cook for 2-3 minutes until just tender.
4. Stir in the pesto sauce and cherry tomatoes.
5. Cook for another 2 minutes until heated through.
6. Season with salt and pepper.
7. Sprinkle with grated Parmesan cheese before serving.

2. Chicken and Avocado Salad

Ingredients:
- 2 cooked chicken breasts, diced
- 1 ripe avocado, diced
- 1 cup mixed greens
- 1/4 cup cherry tomatoes, halved
- 1/4 cup red onion, thinly sliced
- 2 tbsp olive oil
- 1 tbsp lemon juice
- Salt and pepper to taste

Instructions:
1. In a large bowl, combine the diced chicken, avocado, mixed greens, cherry tomatoes, and red onion.
2. Drizzle with olive oil and lemon juice.
3. Toss to combine.
4. Season with salt and pepper.
5. Serve immediately.

3. Cauliflower Fried Rice

Ingredients:
- 1 small head of cauliflower, grated (or 3 cups cauliflower rice)
- 1 cup mixed vegetables (peas, carrots, corn)
- 2 eggs, beaten
- 2 tbsp soy sauce (or coconut aminos)
- 1 tbsp sesame oil
- 2 green onions, sliced
- 1 clove garlic, minced
- Salt and pepper to taste

Instructions:
1. Heat sesame oil in a large skillet or wok over medium heat.
2. Add the garlic and cook until fragrant, about 1 minute.
3. Add the mixed vegetables and cook until tender, about 5 minutes.
4. Push the vegetables to one side of the skillet and pour the beaten eggs into the other side. Scramble the eggs until cooked through.
5. Add the grated cauliflower and soy sauce to the skillet.
6. Stir everything together and cook for another 5 minutes until the cauliflower is tender.
7. Season with salt and pepper.
8. Garnish with sliced green onions before serving.

4. Turkey Lettuce Wraps

Ingredients:
- 1 lb ground turkey
- 1/2 cup diced bell peppers
- 1/2 cup diced onions
- 1 clove garlic, minced
- 2 tbsp soy sauce (or coconut aminos)
- 1 tbsp hoisin sauce (optional)
- 1 head of butter lettuce, leaves separated
- Salt and pepper to taste
- Sliced green onions and sesame seeds for garnish

Instructions:
1. In a large skillet, cook the ground turkey over medium heat until browned, about 5-7 minutes.
2. Add the diced bell peppers, onions, and garlic. Cook until vegetables are tender, about 5 minutes.
3. Stir in the soy sauce and hoisin sauce (if using).
4. Season with salt and pepper.
5. Spoon the turkey mixture into the lettuce leaves.
6. Garnish with sliced green onions and sesame seeds.
7. Serve immediately.

5. Greek Salad with Grilled Chicken

Ingredients:
- 2 cooked chicken breasts, sliced
- 2 cups mixed greens
- 1/2 cup cherry tomatoes, halved
- 1/2 cucumber, sliced
- 1/4 cup red onion, thinly sliced
- 1/4 cup Kalamata olives
- 1/4 cup feta cheese, crumbled
- 2 tbsp olive oil

- 1 tbsp red wine vinegar
- 1 tsp dried oregano
- Salt and pepper to taste

Instructions:
1. In a large bowl, combine the mixed greens, cherry tomatoes, cucumber, red onion, Kalamata olives, and feta cheese.
2. Drizzle with olive oil and red wine vinegar.
3. Sprinkle with dried oregano.
4. Toss to combine.
5. Top with sliced grilled chicken.
6. Season with salt and pepper.
7. Serve immediately.

6. Spinach and Feta Stuffed Chicken Breasts

Ingredients:
- 4 boneless, skinless chicken breasts
- 1 cup fresh spinach, chopped
- 1/2 cup feta cheese, crumbled
- 1 clove garlic, minced
- 1 tbsp olive oil
- Salt and pepper to taste

Instructions:
1. Preheat the oven to 375°F (190°C).
2. In a small bowl, combine the chopped spinach, feta cheese, and minced garlic.
3. Slice a pocket into each chicken breast.
4. Stuff each pocket with the spinach and feta mixture.
5. Secure with toothpicks if necessary.
6. Heat olive oil in a large oven-safe skillet over medium-high heat.
7. Season the chicken breasts with salt and pepper.
8. Sear the chicken breasts for 3-4 minutes on each side until golden brown.
9. Transfer the skillet to the preheated oven and bake for 20-25 minutes until the chicken is cooked through.

10. Serve warm.

7. Eggplant Lasagna

Ingredients:
- 1 large eggplant, sliced lengthwise into 1/4-inch slices
- 1 cup ricotta cheese
- 1 cup shredded mozzarella cheese
- 1/2 cup grated Parmesan cheese
- 1 egg
- 2 cups marinara sauce
- 1 tbsp olive oil
- Salt and pepper to taste
- Fresh basil for garnish

Instructions:
1. Preheat the oven to 375°F (190°C).
2. Arrange the eggplant slices on a baking sheet and brush with olive oil. Season with salt and pepper.
3. Roast the eggplant slices for 20 minutes, until tender.
4. In a bowl, combine the ricotta cheese, half of the mozzarella cheese, Parmesan cheese, and egg. Mix well.
5. In a baking dish, spread a layer of marinara sauce.
6. Layer with eggplant slices, ricotta mixture, and marinara sauce. Repeat layers, ending with marinara sauce.
7. Sprinkle with the remaining mozzarella cheese.
8. Bake for 25-30 minutes until bubbly and golden.
9. Garnish with fresh basil.
10. Serve warm.

8. Shrimp and Avocado Salad

Ingredients:
- 1 lb cooked shrimp, peeled and deveined
- 1 ripe avocado, diced

- 1 cup cherry tomatoes, halved
- 1/4 cup red onion, thinly sliced
- 1 cup mixed greens
- 2 tbsp olive oil
- 1 tbsp lemon juice
- Salt and pepper to taste

Instructions:

1. In a large bowl, combine the cooked shrimp, diced avocado, cherry tomatoes, red onion, and mixed greens.
2. Drizzle with olive oil and lemon juice.
3. Toss to combine.
4. Season with salt and pepper.
5. Serve immediately.

9. Buffalo Cauliflower Bites

Ingredients:

- 1 small head of cauliflower, cut into florets
- 1/4 cup hot sauce
- 2 tbsp melted butter
- 1 tsp garlic powder
- 1 tsp paprika
- Salt and pepper to taste
- Blue cheese or ranch dressing for dipping

Instructions:

1. Preheat the oven to 425°F (220°C).
2. In a bowl, combine the hot sauce, melted butter, garlic powder, paprika, salt, and pepper.
3. Toss the cauliflower florets in the sauce mixture.
4. Arrange the coated cauliflower on a baking sheet lined with parchment paper.
5. Bake for 20-25 minutes until the cauliflower is tender and slightly crispy.
6. Serve with blue cheese or ranch dressing for dipping.

10. Turkey and Spinach Stuffed Bell Peppers

Ingredients:
- 4 large bell peppers (any color)
- 1 lb ground turkey
- 1 cup fresh spinach, chopped
- 1/2 cup diced tomatoes
- 1/2 cup diced onions
- 1 clove garlic, minced
- 1 tbsp olive oil
- 1 tsp Italian seasoning
- Salt and pepper to taste
- 1/2 cup shredded mozzarella cheese (optional)

Instructions:
1. Preheat the oven to 375°F (190°C).
2. Cut the tops off the bell peppers and remove the seeds and membranes.
3. In a large skillet, heat olive oil over medium heat.
4. Add the ground turkey, diced onions, and garlic. Cook until the turkey is browned, about 5-7 minutes.
5. Stir in the chopped spinach, diced tomatoes, Italian seasoning, salt, and pepper. Cook for another 5 minutes until the spinach is wilted.
6. Stuff each bell pepper with the turkey mixture.
7. Place the stuffed peppers in a baking dish.
8. Sprinkle with shredded mozzarella cheese if desired.
9. Cover with foil and bake for 25 minutes. Remove the foil and bake for an additional 10-15 minutes until the peppers are tender.
10. Serve warm.

Low Carb Dinner

1. Garlic Butter Shrimp with Asparagus

Ingredients:
- 1 lb shrimp, peeled and deveined
- 1 bunch asparagus, trimmed and cut into 2-inch pieces
- 3 cloves garlic, minced
- 3 tbsp butter
- 1 tbsp olive oil
- 1 tbsp lemon juice
- Salt and pepper to taste
- Fresh parsley for garnish

Instructions:
1. Heat olive oil in a large skillet over medium heat.
2. Add the asparagus and cook for 3-4 minutes until tender-crisp. Remove and set aside.
3. In the same skillet, add the butter and garlic. Cook for 1-2 minutes until fragrant.
4. Add the shrimp and cook for 2-3 minutes on each side until pink and opaque.
5. Return the asparagus to the skillet and stir to combine.
6. Drizzle with lemon juice and season with salt and pepper.
7. Garnish with fresh parsley before serving.

2. Zucchini Lasagna

Ingredients:
- 2 large zucchinis, sliced lengthwise into thin strips
- 1 lb ground beef
- 1 cup marinara sauce
- 1 cup ricotta cheese
- 1 cup shredded mozzarella cheese
- 1/2 cup grated Parmesan cheese
- 1 egg
- 1 clove garlic, minced

- Salt and pepper to taste
- Fresh basil for garnish

Instructions:
1. Preheat the oven to 375°F (190°C).
2. In a large skillet, cook the ground beef over medium heat until browned. Add the garlic and cook for 1 minute.
3. Stir in the marinara sauce and simmer for 10 minutes.
4. In a bowl, combine the ricotta cheese, egg, and half of the Parmesan cheese. Season with salt and pepper.
5. In a baking dish, spread a layer of meat sauce. Layer with zucchini slices, ricotta mixture, and mozzarella cheese. Repeat layers, ending with meat sauce and remaining mozzarella cheese.
6. Sprinkle with the remaining Parmesan cheese.
7. Bake for 30-35 minutes until bubbly and golden.
8. Garnish with fresh basil before serving.

3. Baked Salmon with Lemon and Dill

Ingredients:
- 4 salmon fillets
- 2 lemons, thinly sliced
- 2 tbsp olive oil
- 2 tbsp fresh dill, chopped
- 2 cloves garlic, minced
- Salt and pepper to taste

Instructions:
1. Preheat the oven to 400°F (200°C).
2. Place the salmon fillets on a baking sheet lined with parchment paper.
3. Drizzle with olive oil and season with salt and pepper.
4. Top each fillet with lemon slices, garlic, and fresh dill.
5. Bake for 15-20 minutes until the salmon is cooked through.
6. Serve with additional lemon slices and dill.

4. Stuffed Bell Peppers

Ingredients:
- 4 large bell peppers (any color)
- 1 lb ground turkey
- 1 cup cauliflower rice
- 1 cup diced tomatoes
- 1/2 cup diced onions
- 1 clove garlic, minced
- 1 tbsp olive oil
- 1 tsp Italian seasoning
- Salt and pepper to taste
- 1/2 cup shredded mozzarella cheese (optional)

Instructions:
1. Preheat the oven to 375°F (190°C).
2. Cut the tops off the bell peppers and remove the seeds and membranes.
3. In a large skillet, heat olive oil over medium heat.
4. Add the ground turkey, diced onions, and garlic. Cook until the turkey is browned, about 5-7 minutes.
5. Stir in the cauliflower rice, diced tomatoes, Italian seasoning, salt, and pepper. Cook for another 5 minutes.
6. Stuff each bell pepper with the turkey mixture.
7. Place the stuffed peppers in a baking dish.
8. Sprinkle with shredded mozzarella cheese if desired.
9. Cover with foil and bake for 25 minutes. Remove the foil and bake for an additional 10-15 minutes until the peppers are tender.
10. Serve warm.

5. Cauliflower Crust Pizza

Ingredients:
- 1 small head of cauliflower, grated (or 3 cups cauliflower rice)
- 1 cup shredded mozzarella cheese
- 1/4 cup grated Parmesan cheese

- 1 egg
- 1 tsp Italian seasoning
- 1/2 cup marinara sauce
- 1 cup shredded mozzarella cheese (for topping)
- 1/4 cup sliced black olives
- 1/4 cup sliced bell peppers
- Salt and pepper to taste

Instructions:
1. Preheat the oven to 425°F (220°C).
2. In a microwave-safe bowl, microwave the grated cauliflower for 5 minutes. Let it cool, then squeeze out excess moisture using a kitchen towel.
3. In a bowl, combine the cauliflower, 1 cup shredded mozzarella cheese, Parmesan cheese, egg, Italian seasoning, salt, and pepper. Mix well.
4. Press the mixture onto a baking sheet lined with parchment paper to form a crust.
5. Bake for 15-20 minutes until golden brown.
6. Spread the marinara sauce over the crust and top with remaining mozzarella cheese, olives, and bell peppers.
7. Bake for an additional 10 minutes until the cheese is melted and bubbly.
8. Serve warm.

6. Chicken Stir-Fry with Broccoli and Bell Peppers

Ingredients:
- 1 lb chicken breast, thinly sliced
- 2 cups broccoli florets
- 1 red bell pepper, sliced
- 1 yellow bell pepper, sliced
- 2 cloves garlic, minced
- 1 tbsp soy sauce (or coconut aminos)
- 1 tbsp sesame oil
- 1 tsp grated ginger
- 1/4 cup chicken broth
- Salt and pepper to taste

- Sesame seeds for garnish

Instructions:
1. Heat sesame oil in a large skillet or wok over medium-high heat.
2. Add the garlic and ginger, and cook until fragrant, about 1 minute.
3. Add the chicken and cook until browned, about 5-7 minutes.
4. Add the broccoli and bell peppers, and stir-fry for another 5 minutes.
5. Stir in the soy sauce and chicken broth.
6. Cook for an additional 3-4 minutes until the vegetables are tender-crisp.
7. Season with salt and pepper.
8. Garnish with sesame seeds before serving.

7. Pork Chops with Creamy Mushroom Sauce

Ingredients:
- 4 boneless pork chops
- 1 cup sliced mushrooms
- 1/2 cup heavy cream
- 1/4 cup chicken broth
- 2 cloves garlic, minced
- 1 tbsp olive oil
- 1 tsp dried thyme
- Salt and pepper to taste
- Fresh parsley for garnish

Instructions:
1. Season the pork chops with salt, pepper, and dried thyme.
2. Heat olive oil in a large skillet over medium-high heat.
3. Add the pork chops and cook for 4-5 minutes on each side until browned and cooked through. Remove and set aside.
4. In the same skillet, add the garlic and mushrooms. Cook for 3-4 minutes until the mushrooms are tender.
5. Stir in the chicken broth and heavy cream.
6. Simmer for 5 minutes until the sauce thickens.
7. Return the pork chops to the skillet and coat with the sauce.

8. Garnish with fresh parsley before serving.

 8. Zoodle Alfredo with Grilled Chicken

Ingredients:
- 2 medium zucchinis, spiralized
- 2 cooked chicken breasts, sliced
- 1 cup heavy cream
- 1/2 cup grated Parmesan cheese
- 2 cloves garlic, minced
- 2 tbsp butter
- Salt and pepper to taste
- Fresh parsley for garnish

Instructions:
1. In a large skillet, melt the butter over medium heat.
2. Add the garlic and cook until fragrant, about 1 minute.
3. Stir in the heavy cream and bring to a simmer.
4. Add the grated Parmesan cheese and cook until the sauce thickens, about 3-4 minutes.
5. Stir in the zucchini noodles and cook for 2-3 minutes until tender.
6. Season with salt and pepper.
7. Top with sliced grilled chicken.
8. Garnish with fresh parsley before serving.

 9. Eggplant Parmesan

Ingredients:
- 1 large eggplant, sliced into 1/4-inch rounds
- 1 cup marinara sauce
- 1 cup shredded mozzarella cheese
- 1/2 cup grated Parmesan cheese
- 1 cup almond flour
- 2 eggs, beaten
- 1 tbsp olive oil

- Salt and pepper to taste
- Fresh basil for garnish

Instructions:
1. Preheat the oven to 375°F (190°C).
2. Season the eggplant slices with salt and pepper.
3. Dip each slice into the beaten eggs, then coat with almond flour.
4. Heat olive oil in a large skillet over medium heat.
5. Fry the eggplant slices for 2-3 minutes on each side until golden brown.
6. In a baking dish, spread a layer of marinara sauce.
7. Layer with fried eggplant slices, marinara sauce, mozzarella cheese, and Parmesan cheese. Repeat layers, ending with cheese.
8. Bake for 25-30 minutes until bubbly and golden.
9. Garnish with fresh basil before serving.

10. Lemon Herb Grilled Chicken Thighs

Ingredients:
- 6 boneless, skinless chicken thighs
- 1/4 cup olive oil
- 2 lemons, juiced
- 3 cloves garlic, minced
- 1 tbsp fresh thyme, chopped
- 1 tbsp fresh rosemary, chopped
- 1 tsp paprika
- Salt and pepper to taste
- Lemon slices for garnish

Instructions:
1. In a bowl, combine olive oil, lemon juice, garlic, thyme, rosemary, paprika, salt, and pepper.
2. Add the chicken thighs to the marinade and toss to coat. Cover and refrigerate for at least 30 minutes.
3. Preheat the grill to medium-high heat.

4. Grill the chicken thighs for 6-7 minutes on each side until cooked through and grill marks appear.
5. Garnish with lemon slices before serving.

Low Carb Snacks and Appetizers

1. Cucumber and Smoked Salmon Bites

Ingredients:
- 1 large cucumber
- 4 oz smoked salmon, thinly sliced
- 4 oz cream cheese, softened
- 1 tbsp fresh dill, chopped
- 1 tbsp lemon juice
- Salt and pepper to taste

Instructions:
1. Slice the cucumber into 1/4-inch rounds.
2. In a bowl, mix the cream cheese, lemon juice, dill, salt, and pepper until smooth.
3. Spread a small amount of the cream cheese mixture onto each cucumber slice.
4. Top with a piece of smoked salmon.
5. Garnish with extra dill if desired.

2. Avocado Deviled Eggs

Ingredients:
- 6 hard-boiled eggs, peeled and halved
- 1 ripe avocado
- 2 tbsp mayonnaise
- 1 tsp Dijon mustard
- 1 tsp lemon juice
- Salt and pepper to taste
- Paprika for garnish

Instructions:
1. Remove the yolks from the halved eggs and place them in a bowl.
2. Add the avocado, mayonnaise, mustard, lemon juice, salt, and pepper to the yolks. Mash until smooth.
3. Spoon or pipe the avocado mixture back into the egg whites.

4. Garnish with a sprinkle of paprika.

3. Cheese and Chive Crackers

Ingredients:
- 1 cup almond flour
- 1 cup shredded cheddar cheese
- 2 tbsp chives, chopped
- 1 egg
- 1/2 tsp salt
- 1/4 tsp garlic powder

Instructions:
1. Preheat the oven to 350°F (175°C).
2. In a bowl, mix the almond flour, cheddar cheese, chives, salt, and garlic powder.
3. Add the egg and mix until a dough forms.
4. Roll the dough out between two sheets of parchment paper to about 1/8-inch thickness.
5. Cut into cracker shapes and place on a baking sheet lined with parchment paper.
6. Bake for 10-12 minutes until golden and crisp.

4. Buffalo Cauliflower Bites

Ingredients:
- 1 head cauliflower, cut into florets
- 1/2 cup almond flour
- 1/2 cup water
- 1/2 tsp garlic powder
- 1/2 tsp onion powder
- 1/2 tsp paprika
- 1/2 tsp salt
- 1/2 cup hot sauce
- 2 tbsp butter, melted

Instructions:
1. Preheat the oven to 425°F (220°C).
2. In a bowl, whisk together the almond flour, water, garlic powder, onion powder, paprika, and salt.
3. Dip each cauliflower floret into the batter, letting the excess drip off.
4. Place on a baking sheet lined with parchment paper and bake for 20 minutes.
5. In a small bowl, mix the hot sauce and melted butter.
6. Toss the baked cauliflower in the hot sauce mixture and return to the oven for another 10 minutes.

5. Spinach and Feta Stuffed Mushrooms

Ingredients:
- 16 large white mushrooms, stems removed
- 1 cup fresh spinach, chopped
- 1/2 cup feta cheese, crumbled
- 1/4 cup cream cheese, softened
- 1 clove garlic, minced
- 1 tbsp olive oil
- Salt and pepper to taste

Instructions:
1. Preheat the oven to 375°F (190°C).
2. In a skillet, heat the olive oil over medium heat.
3. Add the garlic and spinach, and cook until wilted.
4. Remove from heat and mix in the feta cheese and cream cheese. Season with salt and pepper.
5. Stuff each mushroom cap with the spinach mixture.
6. Place on a baking sheet and bake for 20 minutes until the mushrooms are tender.

6. Guacamole and Veggie Sticks

Ingredients:
- 2 ripe avocados
- 1 small tomato, diced

- 1/4 cup red onion, finely chopped
- 1 clove garlic, minced
- 1 tbsp lime juice
- 1 tbsp fresh cilantro, chopped
- Salt and pepper to taste
- Assorted veggie sticks (carrots, celery, bell peppers)

Instructions:
1. In a bowl, mash the avocados with lime juice.
2. Stir in the tomato, red onion, garlic, cilantro, salt, and pepper.
3. Serve with assorted veggie sticks.

7. Prosciutto-Wrapped Asparagus

Ingredients:
- 1 bunch asparagus, trimmed
- 8 slices prosciutto, halved lengthwise
- 1 tbsp olive oil
- Salt and pepper to taste

Instructions:
1. Preheat the oven to 400°F (200°C).
2. Wrap each asparagus spear with a strip of prosciutto.
3. Place on a baking sheet and drizzle with olive oil.
4. Season with salt and pepper.
5. Bake for 15-20 minutes until the asparagus is tender and the prosciutto is crispy.

8. Baked Zucchini Fries

Ingredients:
- 2 large zucchinis, cut into fry shapes
- 1/2 cup almond flour
- 1/2 cup grated Parmesan cheese
- 1 tsp garlic powder
- 1 tsp Italian seasoning

- 1/2 tsp salt
- 1/2 tsp black pepper
- 2 eggs, beaten

Instructions:
1. Preheat the oven to 425°F (220°C).
2. In a bowl, mix the almond flour, Parmesan cheese, garlic powder, Italian seasoning, salt, and pepper.
3. Dip the zucchini fries into the beaten eggs, then coat with the almond flour mixture.
4. Place on a baking sheet lined with parchment paper.
5. Bake for 20-25 minutes until golden and crispy.

9. Caprese Skewers

Ingredients:
- 16 cherry tomatoes
- 16 mini mozzarella balls
- 16 fresh basil leaves
- 2 tbsp balsamic glaze

Instructions:
1. On each skewer, thread a cherry tomato, a basil leaf, and a mozzarella ball.
2. Arrange on a platter and drizzle with balsamic glaze before serving.

10. Tuna Salad Lettuce Wraps

Ingredients:
- 1 can tuna, drained
- 2 tbsp mayonnaise
- 1 tbsp Dijon mustard
- 1 celery stalk, finely chopped
- 1/4 cup red onion, finely chopped
- Salt and pepper to taste
- 8 large lettuce leaves

Instructions:

1. In a bowl, mix the tuna, mayonnaise, Dijon mustard, celery, red onion, salt, and pepper.

2. Spoon the tuna mixture into the center of each lettuce leaf.

3. Roll up the lettuce leaves to form wraps.

Chapter 4: Moderate-Carb Recipes

Moderate Carb Breakfast

1. Berry Smoothie Bowl

Ingredients:
- 1 cup mixed berries (strawberries, blueberries, raspberries)
- 1 banana
- 1/2 cup Greek yogurt
- 1/2 cup almond milk
- 1 tbsp chia seeds
- 1/4 cup granola

Instructions:
1. Blend the mixed berries, banana, Greek yogurt, and almond milk until smooth.
2. Pour into a bowl.
3. Top with chia seeds and granola.

2. Oatmeal with Nuts and Dried Fruit

Ingredients:
- 1/2 cup rolled oats
- 1 cup water or milk
- 1/4 cup mixed nuts (almonds, walnuts, pecans)
- 1/4 cup dried fruit (raisins, cranberries, apricots)
- 1 tbsp honey
- 1/2 tsp cinnamon

Instructions:
1. Cook oats according to package instructions.
2. Stir in honey and cinnamon.
3. Top with mixed nuts and dried fruit.

3. Avocado Toast with Poached Egg

Ingredients:
- 1 slice whole grain bread, toasted
- 1/2 avocado, mashed
- 1 poached egg
- Salt and pepper to taste
- Red pepper flakes (optional)

Instructions:
1. Spread mashed avocado on the toast.
2. Top with the poached egg.
3. Season with salt, pepper, and red pepper flakes if desired.

4. Quinoa Breakfast Bowl

Ingredients:
- 1/2 cup cooked quinoa
- 1/2 cup almond milk
- 1/4 cup fresh berries
- 1 tbsp chopped nuts (almonds, walnuts)
- 1 tbsp honey

Instructions:
1. Warm the cooked quinoa with almond milk.
2. Top with fresh berries, chopped nuts, and honey.

5. Banana Pancakes

Ingredients:
- 1 ripe banana
- 2 eggs
- 1/4 cup rolled oats
- 1/2 tsp baking powder
- 1/4 tsp cinnamon

- 1/4 tsp vanilla extract

Instructions:
1. Blend all ingredients until smooth.
2. Heat a non-stick skillet over medium heat and pour batter to form small pancakes.
3. Cook for 2-3 minutes on each side until golden brown.
4. Serve with fresh fruit or a drizzle of honey.

6. Yogurt Parfait

Ingredients:
- 1 cup Greek yogurt
- 1/2 cup granola
- 1/2 cup mixed berries
- 1 tbsp honey

Instructions:
1. Layer Greek yogurt, granola, and mixed berries in a glass or bowl.
2. Drizzle with honey.

7. Veggie Omelette

Ingredients:
- 2 eggs
- 1/4 cup diced bell peppers
- 1/4 cup diced tomatoes
- 1/4 cup spinach, chopped
- 1/4 cup shredded cheese
- Salt and pepper to taste

Instructions:
1. Whisk the eggs in a bowl.
2. Heat a non-stick skillet over medium heat and add the bell peppers, tomatoes, and spinach. Cook until softened.

3. Pour the eggs over the veggies and cook until the edges start to set.
4. Sprinkle with cheese and fold the omelette in half.
5. Cook until the cheese is melted and the eggs are fully cooked.

8. Sweet Potato Hash

Ingredients:
- 1 large sweet potato, peeled and diced
- 1/2 onion, diced
- 1/2 bell pepper, diced
- 2 tbsp olive oil
- 1 clove garlic, minced
- Salt and pepper to taste

Instructions:
1. Heat olive oil in a skillet over medium heat.
2. Add the sweet potato, onion, bell pepper, and garlic. Cook until the sweet potatoes are tender and slightly crispy.
3. Season with salt and pepper.

9. Cottage Cheese and Fruit

Ingredients:
- 1 cup cottage cheese
- 1/2 cup pineapple chunks
- 1/4 cup blueberries
- 1 tbsp honey

Instructions:
1. Scoop the cottage cheese into a bowl.
2. Top with pineapple chunks, blueberries, and honey.

10. Almond Butter and Banana Sandwich

Ingredients:
- 2 slices whole grain bread
- 2 tbsp almond butter
- 1 banana, sliced
- 1 tbsp chia seeds (optional)

Instructions:
1. Spread almond butter on one slice of bread.
2. Arrange banana slices on top.
3. Sprinkle with chia seeds if desired.
4. Top with the other slice of bread to form a sandwich.

Moderate Carb Lunch

1. Chicken Quinoa Salad

Ingredients:
- 1 cup cooked quinoa
- 1 cup cooked chicken breast, diced
- 1/2 cup cherry tomatoes, halved
- 1/2 cucumber, diced
- 1/4 cup red onion, diced
- 2 tbsp olive oil
- 1 tbsp lemon juice
- Salt and pepper to taste
- Fresh parsley, chopped

Instructions:
1. In a large bowl, combine the quinoa, chicken, cherry tomatoes, cucumber, and red onion.
2. In a small bowl, whisk together the olive oil, lemon juice, salt, and pepper.
3. Pour the dressing over the salad and toss to combine.
4. Garnish with fresh parsley before serving.

2. Turkey and Veggie Wrap

Ingredients:
- 1 whole wheat tortilla
- 3 slices turkey breast
- 1/4 avocado, sliced
- 1/2 cup mixed greens
- 1/4 cup shredded carrots
- 1 tbsp hummus

Instructions:
1. Spread hummus over the tortilla.
2. Layer the turkey, avocado, mixed greens, and shredded carrots on top.

3. Roll up the tortilla tightly and slice in half.

3. Stuffed Bell Peppers

Ingredients:
- 4 bell peppers, tops cut off and seeds removed
- 1 cup cooked brown rice
- 1/2 lb ground turkey
- 1/2 cup diced tomatoes
- 1/2 cup black beans, rinsed and drained
- 1/4 cup corn kernels
- 1/4 cup shredded cheese
- 1 tsp cumin
- Salt and pepper to taste

Instructions:
1. Preheat the oven to 375°F (190°C).
2. In a skillet, cook the ground turkey over medium heat until browned. Drain any excess fat.
3. Add the diced tomatoes, black beans, corn, cumin, salt, and pepper to the skillet. Stir to combine.
4. Stir in the cooked brown rice.
5. Stuff the bell peppers with the mixture and place them in a baking dish.
6. Sprinkle shredded cheese on top of each stuffed pepper.
7. Bake for 25-30 minutes until the peppers are tender and the cheese is melted.

4. Lentil Soup

Ingredients:
- 1 cup lentils, rinsed
- 1 tbsp olive oil
- 1 onion, diced
- 2 carrots, diced
- 2 celery stalks, diced
- 2 cloves garlic, minced

- 6 cups vegetable broth
- 1 can diced tomatoes (14.5 oz)
- 1 tsp cumin
- 1 tsp paprika
- Salt and pepper to taste
- Fresh parsley, chopped

Instructions:
1. Heat olive oil in a large pot over medium heat.
2. Add the onion, carrots, celery, and garlic. Cook until softened.
3. Stir in the cumin and paprika.
4. Add the lentils, vegetable broth, and diced tomatoes. Bring to a boil.
5. Reduce the heat and simmer for 25-30 minutes until the lentils are tender.
6. Season with salt and pepper.
7. Garnish with fresh parsley before serving.

5. Shrimp and Avocado Salad

Ingredients:
- 1/2 lb cooked shrimp, peeled and deveined
- 1 avocado, diced
- 1 cup cherry tomatoes, halved
- 1/2 cucumber, diced
- 2 tbsp olive oil
- 1 tbsp lemon juice
- Salt and pepper to taste
- Fresh dill, chopped

Instructions:
1. In a large bowl, combine the shrimp, avocado, cherry tomatoes, and cucumber.
2. In a small bowl, whisk together the olive oil, lemon juice, salt, and pepper.
3. Pour the dressing over the salad and toss to combine.
4. Garnish with fresh dill before serving.

6. Chickpea and Spinach Stew

Ingredients:
- 1 can chickpeas (15 oz), rinsed and drained
- 1 tbsp olive oil
- 1 onion, diced
- 2 cloves garlic, minced
- 1 can diced tomatoes (14.5 oz)
- 2 cups spinach, chopped
- 1 tsp cumin
- 1 tsp paprika
- Salt and pepper to taste

Instructions:
1. Heat olive oil in a large pot over medium heat.
2. Add the onion and garlic. Cook until softened.
3. Stir in the cumin and paprika.
4. Add the chickpeas and diced tomatoes. Bring to a boil.
5. Reduce the heat and simmer for 10 minutes.
6. Stir in the spinach and cook until wilted.
7. Season with salt and pepper before serving.

7. Whole Wheat Pasta with Pesto and Veggies

Ingredients:
- 2 cups cooked whole wheat pasta
- 1/2 cup cherry tomatoes, halved
- 1/2 cup broccoli florets, steamed
- 1/4 cup pesto sauce
- 2 tbsp grated Parmesan cheese
- Salt and pepper to taste

Instructions:
1. In a large bowl, combine the cooked pasta, cherry tomatoes, and steamed broccoli.

2. Stir in the pesto sauce until well coated.
3. Season with salt and pepper.
4. Sprinkle with grated Parmesan cheese before serving.

8. Tuna Salad Lettuce Wraps

Ingredients:
- 1 can tuna, drained
- 1/4 cup Greek yogurt
- 1 tbsp Dijon mustard
- 1 celery stalk, diced
- 1/4 red onion, diced
- 1 tbsp fresh dill, chopped
- Salt and pepper to taste
- Large lettuce leaves

Instructions:
1. In a bowl, combine the tuna, Greek yogurt, Dijon mustard, celery, red onion, and dill.
2. Season with salt and pepper.
3. Spoon the tuna mixture onto large lettuce leaves and roll up to serve.

9. Chicken and Vegetable Stir-Fry

Ingredients:
- 1 lb chicken breast, sliced into thin strips
- 2 tbsp olive oil
- 1 red bell pepper, sliced
- 1 yellow bell pepper, sliced
- 1 broccoli crown, cut into florets
- 1 carrot, sliced
- 2 cloves garlic, minced
- 2 tbsp soy sauce
- 1 tbsp honey
- 1 tsp sesame oil

Instructions:
1. Heat olive oil in a large skillet over medium-high heat.
2. Add the chicken strips and cook until browned and cooked through. Remove from the skillet and set aside.
3. In the same skillet, add the bell peppers, broccoli, carrot, and garlic. Cook until the vegetables are tender-crisp.
4. Return the chicken to the skillet.
5. Stir in the soy sauce, honey, and sesame oil. Cook for another 2-3 minutes until everything is well coated and heated through.

10. Quinoa and Black Bean Stuffed Sweet Potatoes

Ingredients:
- 2 large sweet potatoes
- 1 cup cooked quinoa
- 1 can black beans (15 oz), rinsed and drained
- 1/2 cup corn kernels
- 1/2 cup diced tomatoes
- 1/4 cup cilantro, chopped
- 1 tbsp lime juice
- Salt and pepper to taste

Instructions:
1. Preheat the oven to 400°F (200°C).
2. Pierce the sweet potatoes with a fork and bake for 45-60 minutes until tender.
3. In a bowl, combine the cooked quinoa, black beans, corn, diced tomatoes, cilantro, lime juice, salt, and pepper.
4. Slice the baked sweet potatoes in half lengthwise and scoop out some of the flesh to create a cavity.
5. Fill the sweet potatoes with the quinoa and black bean mixture.

Moderate Carb Dinner

1. Grilled Salmon with Quinoa and Asparagus

Ingredients:
- 4 salmon fillets
- 1 cup quinoa
- 2 cups water or chicken broth
- 1 bunch asparagus, trimmed
- 2 tbsp olive oil
- 1 lemon, sliced
- Salt and pepper to taste

Instructions:
1. Preheat the grill to medium-high heat.
2. Rinse the quinoa under cold water. Combine quinoa and water (or broth) in a pot, bring to a boil, then reduce to a simmer. Cover and cook for 15 minutes or until water is absorbed.
3. Toss the asparagus with 1 tbsp olive oil, salt, and pepper.
4. Season the salmon fillets with salt and pepper.
5. Grill the salmon for about 4-5 minutes per side until cooked through.
6. Grill the asparagus for about 3-4 minutes, turning occasionally, until tender.
7. Serve the salmon and asparagus over the cooked quinoa, and garnish with lemon slices.

2. Chicken and Vegetable Skewers

Ingredients:
- 1 lb chicken breast, cut into cubes
- 1 red bell pepper, cut into chunks
- 1 yellow bell pepper, cut into chunks
- 1 zucchini, sliced
- 1 red onion, cut into chunks
- 2 tbsp olive oil
- 1 tbsp lemon juice

- 1 tsp garlic powder
- 1 tsp dried oregano
- Salt and pepper to taste
- Wooden skewers (soaked in water for 30 minutes)

Instructions:
1. Preheat the grill to medium-high heat.
2. In a bowl, combine olive oil, lemon juice, garlic powder, oregano, salt, and pepper.
3. Thread the chicken and vegetables onto the skewers.
4. Brush the skewers with the marinade.
5. Grill the skewers for about 10-12 minutes, turning occasionally, until the chicken is cooked through and the vegetables are tender.

3. Stuffed Zucchini Boats
Ingredients:
- 4 medium zucchinis, halved lengthwise and seeds scooped out
- 1 lb ground turkey
- 1 cup diced tomatoes
- 1/2 cup quinoa, cooked
- 1/4 cup diced onion
- 1 tsp garlic powder
- 1 tsp dried oregano
- 1/2 cup shredded mozzarella cheese
- Salt and pepper to taste

Instructions:
1. Preheat the oven to 375°F (190°C).
2. In a skillet, cook the ground turkey with diced onion until browned. Drain any excess fat.
3. Add the diced tomatoes, cooked quinoa, garlic powder, oregano, salt, and pepper to the skillet. Cook for another 2-3 minutes.
4. Stuff the zucchini halves with the turkey mixture and place them in a baking dish.
5. Top with shredded mozzarella cheese.

6. Bake for 20-25 minutes until the zucchini is tender and the cheese is melted and bubbly.

4. Turkey Meatballs with Spaghetti Squash

Ingredients:
- 1 medium spaghetti squash
- 1 lb ground turkey
- 1/4 cup grated Parmesan cheese
- 1/4 cup breadcrumbs
- 1 egg
- 2 cloves garlic, minced
- 1 tsp dried oregano
- 1 tsp dried basil
- Salt and pepper to taste
- 1 jar marinara sauce

Instructions:
1. Preheat the oven to 400°F (200°C).
2. Cut the spaghetti squash in half, remove seeds, and bake cut-side down on a baking sheet for 40-45 minutes until tender.
3. In a bowl, combine the ground turkey, Parmesan cheese, breadcrumbs, egg, garlic, oregano, basil, salt, and pepper. Mix well.
4. Form the mixture into meatballs and place them on a baking sheet.
5. Bake the meatballs for 20-25 minutes until cooked through.
6. Heat the marinara sauce in a pot and add the cooked meatballs.
7. Use a fork to scrape the flesh of the spaghetti squash into strands.
8. Serve the meatballs over the spaghetti squash and top with marinara sauce.

5. Chicken Fajita Bowl

Ingredients:
- 1 lb chicken breast, sliced
- 1 red bell pepper, sliced
- 1 yellow bell pepper, sliced

- 1 onion, sliced
- 1 tbsp olive oil
- 1 tsp chili powder
- 1 tsp cumin
- 1/2 tsp paprika
- 1/2 tsp garlic powder
- 1 cup cooked brown rice
- 1/2 cup black beans, rinsed and drained
- 1/2 cup corn kernels
- 1/4 cup salsa
- 1/4 cup shredded cheese
- Salt and pepper to taste

Instructions:
1. Heat olive oil in a skillet over medium-high heat.
2. Add the chicken, bell peppers, and onion. Cook until the chicken is cooked through and the vegetables are tender.
3. Season with chili powder, cumin, paprika, garlic powder, salt, and pepper.
4. In a bowl, layer the brown rice, black beans, corn, chicken, and vegetables.
5. Top with salsa and shredded cheese before serving.

6. Baked Cod with Roasted Vegetables

Ingredients:
- 4 cod fillets
- 1 tbsp olive oil
- 1 lemon, sliced
- 1 tsp garlic powder
- 1 tsp dried thyme
- 2 cups mixed vegetables (e.g., carrots, broccoli, bell peppers), chopped
- Salt and pepper to taste

Instructions:
1. Preheat the oven to 375°F (190°C).
2. Place the cod fillets on a baking sheet lined with parchment paper.

3. Drizzle with olive oil and sprinkle with garlic powder, thyme, salt, and pepper.
4. Arrange lemon slices on top of the cod.
5. Spread the mixed vegetables around the cod on the baking sheet.
6. Bake for 20-25 minutes until the cod is cooked through and the vegetables are tender.

7. Beef and Broccoli Stir-Fry

Ingredients:
- 1 lb flank steak, thinly sliced
- 1 head broccoli, cut into florets
- 2 tbsp soy sauce
- 1 tbsp oyster sauce
- 1 tbsp hoisin sauce
- 1 tbsp cornstarch
- 2 cloves garlic, minced
- 1 tbsp ginger, minced
- 2 tbsp vegetable oil
- 1/2 cup beef broth
- Cooked brown rice, for serving

Instructions:
1. In a bowl, combine soy sauce, oyster sauce, hoisin sauce, and cornstarch.
2. Heat 1 tbsp vegetable oil in a skillet over medium-high heat. Add the beef and cook until browned. Remove and set aside.
3. In the same skillet, heat the remaining oil. Add garlic, ginger, and broccoli. Cook until the broccoli is tender-crisp.
4. Return the beef to the skillet and pour in the sauce mixture and beef broth. Cook until the sauce thickens.
5. Serve over cooked brown rice.

8. Vegetable and Chickpea Curry

Ingredients:
- 1 tbsp olive oil

- 1 onion, diced
- 2 cloves garlic, minced
- 1 tbsp ginger, minced
- 1 tbsp curry powder
- 1 tsp turmeric
- 1 can diced tomatoes (14.5 oz)
- 1 can coconut milk (14 oz)
- 1 can chickpeas (15 oz), rinsed and drained
- 2 cups mixed vegetables (e.g., bell peppers, carrots, peas), chopped
- Fresh cilantro, chopped
- Cooked brown rice or quinoa, for serving

Instructions:
1. Heat olive oil in a large pot over medium heat.
2. Add the onion, garlic, and ginger. Cook until softened.
3. Stir in the curry powder and turmeric.
4. Add the diced tomatoes and coconut milk. Bring to a simmer.
5. Stir in the chickpeas and mixed vegetables. Cook until the vegetables are tender.
6. Serve over cooked brown rice or quinoa, garnished with fresh cilantro.

9. Pesto Chicken with Zucchini Noodles

Ingredients:
- 4 chicken breasts
- 1 cup pesto sauce
- 4 zucchinis, spiralized into noodles
- 1 tbsp olive oil
- 1/4 cup grated Parmesan cheese
- Salt and pepper to taste

Instructions:
1. Preheat the oven to 375°F (190°C).
2. Place the chicken breasts in a baking dish and spread pesto sauce over each breast.

3. Bake for 25-30 minutes until the chicken is cooked through.
4. In a skillet, heat olive oil over medium heat. Add the zucchini noodles and cook for 2-3 minutes until tender.
5. Serve the pesto chicken over the zucchini noodles and top with grated Parmesan cheese.

10. Turkey and Sweet Potato Skillet

Ingredients:
- 1 lb ground turkey
- 2 medium sweet potatoes, peeled and diced
- 1 onion, diced
- 1 bell pepper, diced
- 2 cloves garlic, minced
- 1 tsp paprika
- 1 tsp cumin
- 1/2 tsp chili powder
- Salt and pepper to taste
- Fresh cilantro, chopped

Instructions:
1. Heat a large skillet over medium-high heat and add the ground turkey. Cook untilcooked through and browned. Remove and set aside.

2. In the same skillet, add the diced sweet potatoes. Cook for about 5-7 minutes until they begin to soften.
3. Add the onion, bell pepper, and garlic to the skillet. Cook for another 3-4 minutes until the vegetables are tender.
4. Return the cooked ground turkey to the skillet.
5. Season with paprika, cumin, chili powder, salt, and pepper. Stir to combine.
6. Cook for an additional 2-3 minutes to allow the flavors to meld.
7. Garnish with fresh cilantro before serving.

Moderate Carb Snacks and Appetizers

1. Greek Yogurt with Berries and Almonds

Ingredients:
- 1 cup Greek yogurt
- 1/2 cup mixed berries (e.g., strawberries, blueberries, raspberries)
- 2 tbsp sliced almonds
- 1 tbsp honey (optional)

Instructions:
1. Spoon Greek yogurt into a bowl or parfait glass.
2. Top with mixed berries and sliced almonds.
3. Drizzle with honey if desired.

2. Cottage Cheese and Pineapple

Ingredients:
- 1 cup cottage cheese
- 1/2 cup diced pineapple

Instructions:
1. Place cottage cheese in a bowl.
2. Top with diced pineapple.
3. Serve chilled.

3. Caprese Skewers

Ingredients:
- Cherry tomatoes
- Fresh mozzarella balls
- Fresh basil leaves
- Balsamic glaze (optional)

Instructions:

1. Thread cherry tomatoes, mozzarella balls, and basil leaves onto skewers.
2. Drizzle with balsamic glaze if desired.

4. Turkey and Cheese Roll-Ups

Ingredients:
- Slices of deli turkey
- Slices of cheese (e.g., cheddar, Swiss)
- Spinach leaves
- Mustard or mayonnaise (optional)

Instructions:
1. Lay a slice of turkey flat.
2. Place a slice of cheese on top.
3. Add a few spinach leaves.
4. Roll up tightly.
5. Secure with a toothpick if needed.
6. Optional: Serve with mustard or mayonnaise for dipping.

5. Avocado and Tomato Slices

Ingredients:
- 1 avocado, sliced
- 1 tomato, sliced
- Salt and pepper to taste

Instructions:
1. Arrange avocado and tomato slices on a plate.
2. Season with salt and pepper.

6. Stuffed Bell Pepper Halves

Ingredients:
- Bell peppers, halved and seeded
- Hummus

- Sliced cucumbers
- Cherry tomatoes, halved

Instructions:
1. Spread hummus inside each bell pepper half.
2. Top with sliced cucumbers and cherry tomato halves.

7. Hard-Boiled Eggs with Guacamole

Ingredients:
- Hard-boiled eggs, sliced in half
- Guacamole

Instructions:
1. Spread guacamole on each egg half.
2. Sprinkle with a pinch of salt and pepper.

8. Edamame with Sea Salt

Ingredients:
- Edamame, steamed
- Sea salt

Instructions:
1. Steam edamame according to package instructions.
2. Sprinkle with sea salt.

9. Mozzarella and Tomato Salad

Ingredients:
- Fresh mozzarella, sliced
- Sliced tomatoes
- Fresh basil leaves
- Balsamic vinegar
- Olive oil

- Salt and pepper to taste

Instructions:
1. Arrange mozzarella slices and tomato slices on a plate.
2. Top with fresh basil leaves.
3. Drizzle with balsamic vinegar and olive oil.
4. Season with salt and pepper.

 10. Tuna Salad Cucumber Bites

Ingredients:
- Cucumber, sliced into rounds
- Tuna salad (canned tuna mixed with mayonnaise or Greek yogurt, diced celery, and seasonings)

Instructions:
1. Place cucumber rounds on a serving platter.
2. Spoon a small amount of tuna salad onto each cucumber round.

Chapter 5: Exercise and Carb Cycling

14 days Meal Plan

Week 1

Day 1 - High Carb
- **Breakfast**: Oatmeal with berries and honey
- **Lunch**: Quinoa salad with chickpeas, cucumber, tomatoes, and feta
- **Dinner**: Grilled chicken with sweet potatoes and steamed broccoli
- **Snack**: Apple slices with almond butter

Day 2 - Low Carb
- **Breakfast**: Spinach and feta omelet
- **Lunch**: Grilled salmon salad with mixed greens, avocado, and olive oil dressing
- **Dinner**: Zucchini noodles with pesto and grilled shrimp
- **Snack**: Greek yogurt with a few almonds

Day 3 - Moderate Carb
- **Breakfast**: Smoothie with banana, spinach, protein powder, and almond milk
- **Lunch**: Turkey and avocado wrap in a whole wheat tortilla
- **Dinner**: Stir-fried tofu with mixed vegetables and brown rice
- **Snack**: Carrot sticks with hummus

Day 4 - High Carb
- **Breakfast**: Whole grain toast with avocado and poached eggs
- **Lunch**: Lentil soup with whole grain crackers
- **Dinner**: Baked salmon with quinoa and roasted vegetables
- **Snack**: Fresh fruit salad

Day 5 - Low Carb
- **Breakfast**: Cottage cheese with blueberries and chia seeds
- **Lunch**: Chicken Caesar salad (no croutons)
- **Dinner**: Beef stir-fry with broccoli and bell peppers

- **Snack**: Celery sticks with peanut butter

Day 6 - Moderate Carb
- **Breakfast**: Greek yogurt parfait with granola and mixed berries
- **Lunch**: Tuna salad with whole grain crackers
- **Dinner**: Spaghetti squash with marinara sauce and turkey meatballs
- **Snack**: Hard-boiled egg and a small apple

Day 7 - High Carb
- **Breakfast**: Pancakes made with whole grain flour and topped with fresh fruit
- **Lunch**: Chickpea and vegetable curry with brown rice
- **Dinner**: Grilled chicken fajitas with whole wheat tortillas, peppers, and onions
- **Snack**: Banana with a handful of nuts

Week 2

Day 8 - Low Carb
- **Breakfast**: Smoked salmon and avocado on a bed of arugula
- **Lunch**: Beef and vegetable stir-fry
- **Dinner**: Grilled pork chops with cauliflower mash and green beans
- **Snack**: Cherry tomatoes and mozzarella balls

Day 9 - Moderate Carb
- **Breakfast**: Overnight oats with chia seeds and mixed berries
- **Lunch**: Whole grain wrap with grilled chicken, lettuce, and hummus
- **Dinner**: Baked cod with quinoa and steamed asparagus
- **Snack**: Sliced bell peppers with guacamole

Day 10 - High Carb
- **Breakfast**: Whole grain cereal with almond milk and banana slices
- **Lunch**: Black bean and corn salad with avocado
- **Dinner**: Whole wheat pasta with marinara sauce and turkey sausage
- **Snack**: Pear slices with cheese

Day 11 - Low Carb

- **Breakfast**: Eggs scrambled with spinach, tomatoes, and cheese
- **Lunch**: Grilled shrimp Caesar salad
- **Dinner**: Baked chicken thighs with roasted Brussels sprouts and carrots
- **Snack**: Almonds and a few berries

Day 12 - Moderate Carb

- **Breakfast**: Protein smoothie with banana, spinach, and almond butter
- **Lunch**: Quinoa and vegetable stuffed bell peppers
- **Dinner**: Turkey chili with a side of whole grain bread
- **Snack**: Greek yogurt with honey and walnuts

Day 13 - High Carb

- **Breakfast**: Whole grain waffles with fresh berries and maple syrup
- **Lunch**: Falafel wrap with tzatziki sauce and a side salad
- **Dinner**: Grilled steak with baked potato and mixed vegetables
- **Snack**: Apple slices with peanut butter

Day 14 - Low Carb

- **Breakfast**: Omelet with mushrooms, bell peppers, and cheese
- **Lunch**: Chicken and avocado salad
- **Dinner**: Grilled salmon with sautéed spinach and zucchini
- **Snack**: Cottage cheese with a few slices of cucumber

Aligning Diet with Workouts

1. High Carb Days and Intense Workouts: On days when you have high-intensity workouts scheduled, such as weightlifting sessions or high-intensity interval training (HIIT), it's beneficial to consume more carbohydrates. Carbohydrates are your body's preferred source of energy for intense physical activities. They replenish glycogen stores in your muscles, which can help you perform better and recover faster.

- Example: Plan high carb days on days when you have leg day at the gym or a HIIT session scheduled. Aim to consume complex carbohydrates like whole grains, sweet potatoes, and fruits to sustain your energy levels throughout your workout.

2. Moderate Carb Days and Moderate Workouts: On moderate workout days, such as moderate cardio sessions or yoga, moderate carbohydrate intake can support your energy needs without overwhelming your system with too many carbs.

   - Example: Choose whole grains like quinoa or brown rice, along with lean proteins and plenty of vegetables. These carbs will provide sustained energy for your workouts without causing a spike in blood sugar levels.

3. Low Carb Days and Rest Days: On rest days or days with light physical activity, lower carbohydrate intake can help your body burn fat more efficiently. Since your energy expenditure is lower, you don't need as many carbs to fuel your activities.

   - Example: Focus on consuming more healthy fats, lean proteins, and fibrous vegetables on low carb days. These nutrients support muscle repair and growth while keeping your overall calorie intake in check.

Planning Your Carb Cycling Schedule

- Personalization: Adjust your carb cycling schedule based on your personal fitness goals, body composition, and workout intensity. Experiment with different ratios of high, moderate, and low carb days to find what works best for you.

- Timing: Plan your meals around your workout schedule. Eat a balanced meal containing protein, carbs, and fats about 1-2 hours before your workout to ensure you have enough energy to perform optimally. After your workout, consume a meal rich in protein and carbohydrates to support muscle recovery and glycogen replenishment.

- Hydration: Stay hydrated throughout your carb cycling plan, as proper hydration is crucial for overall performance and recovery.

Monitoring Progress and Adjustments

- Listen to Your Body: Pay attention to how your body responds to different carb cycling patterns and adjust accordingly. You may need to tweak the timing or composition of your meals based on your energy levels, hunger cues, and fitness progress.

- Consultation: Consider consulting with a nutritionist or fitness coach who specializes in carb cycling to help you create a personalized plan that aligns with your fitness goals and lifestyle.

By aligning your diet with your workouts through carb cycling, you can optimize your energy levels, improve performance, and achieve your fitness goals more effectively.

Chapter 6: Overcoming Challenges

Carb cycling can be an effective strategy for achieving your fitness and weight loss goals, but it also comes with its own set of challenges. Understanding these challenges and learning how to overcome them is key to maintaining consistency and success in your carb cycling journey.

Common Pitfalls

1. Overly Restrictive Low Carb Days: One common pitfall is making low carb days too restrictive, which can lead to feelings of deprivation and make it difficult to stick with the plan long-term. It's important to include enough variety and nutrients on low carb days to keep you satisfied and prevent binge eating later.

   - Solution: Include plenty of non-starchy vegetables, lean proteins, and healthy fats on low carb days. This will help you feel full and satisfied while still keeping your carbohydrate intake low.

2. Inconsistency: Another challenge is inconsistency in following the carb cycling schedule. Life can be unpredictable, and it's easy to skip or modify planned high or low carb days.

   - Solution: Plan ahead and schedule your high, moderate, and low carb days based on your weekly routine. Prepare meals in advance and have healthy snacks on hand to stay on track, even during busy days.

3. Lack of Planning: Not planning your meals and snacks ahead of time can lead to making poor food choices, especially when cravings strike.

   - Solution: Create a meal plan for each week that includes a variety of foods for high, moderate, and low carb days. Prepare meals in bulk when possible and pack snacks to take with you when you're on the go.

4. Social Pressures: Social gatherings and events can often present challenges, as they may involve high carb foods and drinks that are not part of your carb cycling plan.

   - Solution: Plan ahead by eating a balanced meal before attending social events. Bring a healthy dish to share that fits within your carb cycling guidelines. Focus on enjoying the company rather than just the food.

Dealing with Cravings

1. Understanding Cravings: Cravings for high carb foods can be triggered by stress, emotions, or habits developed over time. Recognizing the difference between hunger and cravings is important for managing them effectively.

   - Solution: Practice mindful eating and listen to your body's hunger cues. If you experience a craving, try distracting yourself with a healthy activity or snack that aligns with your carb cycling plan.

2. Healthy Substitutions: Instead of giving in to unhealthy cravings, find healthier alternatives that still satisfy your taste buds without derailing your progress.

   - Example: Replace sugary snacks with fresh fruit or Greek yogurt with berries. Choose air-popped popcorn or nuts instead of chips.

3. Moderation: Allow yourself small indulgences occasionally to prevent feelings of deprivation. Incorporate your favorite foods in moderation and adjust your carb cycling schedule accordingly.

   - Example: Plan a high carb day around a special occasion or treat yourself to a small portion of your favorite dessert without guilt.

Staying Motivated

1. Setting Realistic Goals: Keep your goals realistic and achievable. Celebrate small victories along the way to stay motivated and committed to your carb cycling plan.

2. Tracking Progress: Monitor your progress by keeping track of your workouts, measurements, and how you feel overall. Seeing tangible results can boost motivation and keep you focused on your goals.

3. Seeking Support: Surround yourself with a supportive network of friends, family, or online communities who can encourage you and provide accountability during your carb cycling journey.

Chapter 7: Tracking Progress

Tracking your progress is crucial in any fitness and nutrition plan, including carb cycling. By monitoring and adjusting your approach, you can ensure that you're moving towards your goals effectively and making necessary tweaks along the way.

Monitoring Progress

1. Measurement Tools: Use various tools to track your progress, such as:
   - Body Measurements: Track changes in inches around key areas like waist, hips, and thighs.
   - Body Weight: Regularly weigh yourself under consistent conditions, such as in the morning after using the restroom.
   - Progress Photos: Take photos from different angles to visually track changes in your body composition.
   - Fitness Assessments: Measure improvements in strength, endurance, and flexibility through fitness tests.

2. Food Journaling: Keep a detailed food journal to record what you eat on high, moderate, and low carb days. This helps you identify patterns, track your calorie intake, and assess how different foods affect your energy levels and cravings.

3. Energy Levels and Mood: Pay attention to how you feel throughout the day. Note any changes in energy levels, mood, and mental clarity, which can provide insights into how well your carb cycling plan is working for you.

Adjusting Your Approach

1. Review and Reflect: Regularly review your progress data and reflect on what's working well and what needs adjustment.

2. Consultation: Consider consulting with a nutritionist, dietitian, or fitness coach who specializes in carb cycling. They can provide personalized guidance based on your progress and help you make informed adjustments to your plan.

3. Tweaking Macronutrient Ratios: Based on your progress and goals, adjust the ratios of high, moderate, and low carb days. Fine-tune the amount and types of carbohydrates, proteins, and fats to optimize your results.

4. Plateaus and Challenges: Address plateaus by incorporating changes such as increasing exercise intensity, trying new recipes, or varying your carb cycling schedule.

Staying Motivated

1. Celebrate Achievements: Celebrate your milestones, whether it's reaching a weight loss goal, improving fitness performance, or sticking to your carb cycling plan consistently.

2. Visualization: Visualize your goals and the benefits of achieving them. Use positive affirmations and visualization techniques to stay motivated and focused on your journey.

3. Accountability: Share your goals and progress with a supportive friend, family member, or online community. Accountability can help you stay committed and motivated during challenging times.

Long-Term Sustainability

1. Lifestyle Integration: Aim for a carb cycling approach that fits your lifestyle and preferences. Sustainable changes are more likely to lead to long-term success.

2. Adaptability: Be adaptable and willing to adjust your carb cycling plan as your goals and circumstances change over time.

3. Reflection and Learning: Continuously learn from your experiences and adjust your approach based on what you discover works best for your body and lifestyle.

Conclusion

Congratulations on completing your journey through the world of carb cycling! Throughout this book, you've learned how to harness the power of carbohydrates to fuel your workouts, optimize your metabolism, and achieve your fitness goals. As you reflect on your carb cycling experience, here's a recap and some final words of encouragement to keep you motivated on your health and wellness journey.

Recap

In this book, you've explored:

- The Basics of Carb Cycling: Understanding the principles of high, moderate, and low carb days and how they can be tailored to your goals and lifestyle.
- Benefits of Carb Cycling: From improving energy levels and enhancing workout performance to supporting fat loss and muscle retention.
- Overcoming Challenges: Strategies for managing cravings, navigating social situations, and staying consistent with your carb cycling plan.
- Tracking Progress: Monitoring your body measurements, energy levels, and food intake to assess your progress and make necessary adjustments.
- Aligning Diet with Exercise: How to synchronize your nutrition with your workouts to maximize results and recovery.

Final Words of Encouragement

As you continue your carb cycling journey, remember:

- Consistency is Key: Stay consistent with your carb cycling plan to see long-term results. Trust the process and be patient with yourself.
- Listen to Your Body: Pay attention to how different foods and carb cycling patterns affect your energy levels, mood, and overall well-being.
- Celebrate Your Successes: Celebrate every milestone and achievement, no matter how small. Each step forward is a step closer to your ultimate health and fitness goals.

- Stay Educated and Adapt: Keep learning about nutrition, fitness, and wellness. Adapt your carb cycling approach as needed to suit your evolving goals and lifestyle.

By incorporating carb cycling into your lifestyle, you've empowered yourself with a versatile tool for achieving and maintaining your desired physique and overall health. Whether your goal is weight loss, muscle gain, or improved athletic performance, carb cycling can support you on your journey towards a healthier, stronger you.

Thank you for joining me on this carb cycling adventure. Here's to your continued success and well-being!